WAKE UP
AND EAT
THE KALE

Produced by:

FriesenPress

Suite 300 – 852 Fort Street

Victoria, BC, Canada V8W 1H8

www.friesenpress.com

Distributed to the trade by The Ingram Book Company

The Flame of Hope is a symbol that burns continuously in Sir Frederick Banting Square in Ontario, Canada. I would like to personally extend this message of hope to all the people of the world who are experiencing their own journey through cancer or any other serious illness.

Wendy M Banting

Table of Contents

WAKE UP AND EAT THE KALE

How I Healed Myself Naturally from Advanced Cancer Using Body, Mind and Spirit

WENDY MARIE BANTING

Introduction

The author makes no claims that anyone who follows her healing regime will be cured. This is due to the many choices and emotional states that vary from person to person over which she has no control. The author takes no responsibility for the outcomes that will be experienced differently for each person. The author seeks only to share her experience and outcomes for the inspiration around her particular success.

My name is Wendy Banting, and I am 54 years old. I was diagnosed with Stage III breast cancer and was told that my chances of being cured from this type of cancer were slim even with the use of chemotherapy, radiation and surgery. Now, three years later, I am still here having lived through a time of self-healing that used neither chemotherapy, radiation nor surgery, but a regime of natural, holistic and spiritual practices. This book is about my healing.

This book is organized into two parts. The first part lists all the natural healing methods I used, including practical knowledge related to diet and physical methods. The second part of the book is about my spiritual journey which, in combination with the practical healing, afforded me my success. This book is designed to help anyone who has disease in any form, whether it be cancer, heart disease or any form of supposed incurable illness. I have laid it out so you can follow my own progression in the order in which I lived it. Be fearless in your courage and determination to be sovereign unto yourselves. Be kind to yourself as you travel your road. It's been my experience that you can cure yourself of anything if you believe you can.

This is a journey of awakening to the presence of body, mind and spirit. I am consciousness inhabiting a body for the purpose of experiencing physical life. I am not the body. Through my journey of healing, I am remembering that I AM.

Foreword

My decision to write a book around my healing journey through cancer began mostly as a desire to impart to others the details and methods I used to successfully heal myself from advanced aggressive breast cancer. For regardless of what any person may think of what I have done, or the way I have done it, I have been successful. I am objective evidence. It might be helpful to keep that in mind as you delve into my story, for at times many things I have written about will seem unbelievable to you. I have looked into the face of the most fearful illness on the planet and stared it down using will, intention, determination, discipline, and ultimately, surrender.

I would like to stress that this is my story, my healing journey, and it is for you, the reader, to take from it what you feel fits with your life, your story. Because each of us are unique pieces in the tapestry of humanity, your highest authority is yourself, and your journey will not be quite the same as mine. You will not have to do all the things I have done or use all of the methods I have used. Your path will unfold in perfection for your experience. Therefore, please take and use any healing modalities or words of wisdom that I have experienced and imparted to you and use them for your own purposes. In the same breath, I would like you to keep in mind that you do not have to do anything that I have done or written that does not resonate with you. It need not be for you. Discernment of what is appropriate for your path is an important part of anyone's journey through life. Listen to your own intuition about what I have written.

There are many reasons why I decided to write this book. And the reasons changed and evolved during the writing of it. Many breaks took place while I was bringing it all forward, and I now understand that these were necessary as each new experience afforded me a more expanded view of the overall journey. The human journey is one of evolvement and expansion. We never get it done. We are always moving to new levels of awareness through our choices and actions. This book you will read is about my story, my journey, my choices which resulted in my actions and ultimately, my truth. It is, on the surface, a story of healing, a journey through the experience of cancer, yet at the end of the day, it is also an adventure into the world of self discovery. It is about the meeting of myself at the soul level and an understanding of the truth of the self that I am here to be. It follows the unveiling of my illusion of who I was and the development into the new human I am meant to be.

All illness is merely emotional growth that everyone goes through in their quest to discover new levels of who they are. It is the soul's way of moving you in the direction of the higher levels of awareness that you are. The fear of going there is what actually creates the physical blockages termed illness, and your resistance to moving into these new levels is what keeps you in a state of disease. Moving from a state of fearing your body, into a state of loving your body, is the real overarching story that I wish to impart to you. So it will be up to you to decide how much you can move out of the limiting thoughts of today's world and move into the courageous limitless arena of the heart and soul, and create a new healthy environment for your thoughts and feelings, and ultimately, create a new reality that resides in health, joy, love and expansion. I honor your journey.

Part 1:

TRADITIONAL MEDICINE VER-SUS HOLISTIC MEDICINE

I chose to heal myself of cancer using primarily holistic medical prac-tices, energy medicine, and a host of other healing modalities that fall under those umbrellas. I chose to listen to my own intuition around what felt right for me. This does not mean that there are not other routes to success. However, the success of any healing regime lies in the letting go of fear. I will say that my choices gave me the best outcome I could have hoped for—I have never felt sick for a day since my diagnosis. I never had any severe pain or the associated physical trauma that usually comes with those who choose surgery, chemotherapy and radiation. But I have known people who have gone that route, and survived, so who is to say that was not the best choice for them? It is everyone's right to choose their own fate, and I offer my experience in the hopes that those who feel compelled to make their own decisions can do so with hope and absolute clarity that another method is not only possible but can be successful in a way that leaves out much of the physical anguish and affords a better quality of life as you move forward. It is imperative that a person *believe* in their own power to heal themselves. I would also like to stress that those who feel compelled to choose chemotherapy, radiation or surgery can still use many of the healing modalities I have used in conjunction with their therapy, but would strongly recommend that they see a naturopathic doctor for help with combining supplements and their medications as prescribed by their traditional doctors. This will give you a tremendous leg up in your recovery.

Chapter 1.
THE DIAGNOSIS

In early April of 2010, I was biopsied for breast cancer at the hospital in Halifax, Nova Scotia, in Canada. The results of that biopsy, which I only looked at recently, showed that I had endocrine sensitive (estrogen and progesterone receptor positive) and HER-2/neu positive locally advanced left breast carcinoma. Quite a mouthful, and I admit that none of that made sense to me either. I did Google the whole thing, and in doing so, was quite pleased that I had not done so earlier in my journey, because while I did know that I was playing with my life in my decision to heal myself, I am not quite sure I realized how dismal the odds were of surviving this form of cancer in the beginning.

That is the technical medical terminology for what type of cancer I had. I discussed this with my oncologist for the purpose of writing this book, and received a layman's interpretation of this diagnosis, which was also reviewed by my oncologist so that I could be assured of the accuracy of the information I am imparting to the reader.

I was told in the beginning that, due to the severity of my cancer, I would need chemotherapy and radiation in order to first shrink the large tumor in my breast that was attached to the skin. This would be followed by surgery if the first two could shrink it enough. This was the established protocol for this sort of cancer. They also tested the cancer to see if it would respond to the drug tamoxifen, and the results showed that it would. I declined all treatment except for the tamoxifen. The following interpretation of the odds of me curing my cancer with just tamoxifen and my holistic approach was given to me by my oncologist.

At the time I was diagnosed by the medical community in Nova Scotia, I was considered a Stage III cancer, and the only reason I was not considered Stage IV by them was because the cancer had not travelled to any other areas in my body. As you will read later in the book, prior to getting my biopsy results, I had travelled to the Philippines to see Jun Labo, a psychic surgeon, who told me I had breast cancer and that it was traveling throughout my body and that he would remove what he termed the *streamers*. Since I did not have any medical testing in Canada until after I came back from the Philippines, they have no evidence of it having travelled. I had various tests when I arrived home, and they came back clear. My oncologist actually stated to me, in the second year of my recovery, that he has never seen my particular cancer eventually not spread. This statement seems to validate the removal of the streamers from Jun Labo.

Due to the rather large size of the cancer in the breast and its firm attachment to the skin, it was deemed to be a more severe situation. The percentage of people who have used only tamoxifen to treat this cancer has a response rate of between ten to fifteen percent, and usually only for a period of one year. So, a low chance at best. The type of cancer that I had is one that is very aggressive in its growth, a gene that turns on and does not turn off, so to speak, and I was in a more advanced state of this disease. My oncologist told me that he really has no scientific under-standing of what I have done to affect the stable form of healing that I present with at this time, three years later, and that my success is highly unusual and remarkable. The odds of surviving this cancer were not that high even with the chemotherapy, radiation and surgery, so my having done so without any of these is a testament to the ability of a person to engage in their own healing and be successful. The way in which I went about this is described in this book, and I want to stress that it is important to read all that I have done, and understand both the physical and spiritual philosophies that I employed, so as to have the optimum outcomes. I cannot take any responsibility for outcomes that individuals may experience, as everyone will have a different journey, and make different choices. All I can state is that this is what I did, and my outcome is very successful, and I wish to share it with the world at large.

I have great appreciation for my oncologist and his sincere desire to help me. I did not give him much space to apply his methodologies and treatment, and while he certainly did not, at the time, understand my decision to heal myself naturally, he was always open-minded and very respectful of my right to do it my way. I came to enjoy the visits, and thank him sincerely for his warm integrity and professionalism.

Chapter 2.
THE BIOLOGY OF THE BODY

The first thing I did was clean up my body. It is important to understand that the immune system is pretty depleted by the time a serious illness engages, and while it may seem like I did a LOT as you read the list of things I have done, it's simply a regime that takes the toxins out of the body and then supports the immune system so it can do its job.

Most people living in our modern world are eating dead food, drinking dead water, and polluting their bodies with poisons, chemicals and pesticides, not to mention all the airborne pollutants. Electrical and microwave frequencies also mess up body rhythms.

Epsom Salt Cleanse

I started with an Epsom salt cleanse. This is pretty simple and yields amazing results. An Epsom salt solution is known scientifically as a *hyper-osmotic*. Just like other salts, Epsom salts attract water, so when Epsom salts are passing through your bowels, the salts pull water from other parts of your body. This makes your digestive system more lubricated, and in turn you will excrete more.

One of the most common side effects of an Epsom salt cleanse is dehydration. Keep this in mind during a cleanse, and drink plenty of water. Other side effects are related to the intestinal tract, so you may experience cramps or gas while doing the cleanse. You can find more information online as to which form of Epsom salt cleanse you want to try. I used 1 teaspoon in 1 cup of warm water daily for two weeks. Check with your doctor first to make sure it is appropriate for you.

The reason I started with the Epsom salt cleanse is that it not only removes built up toxic waste from the colon, it also removes it from the small and large intestines. This is why colonics are not my preferred method—the intestines get overlooked. If you start any detoxification practice without doing an Epsom salt cleanse first, any purifying efforts that you make will be filtering through the existing dirty condition of your elimination system. I will warn you, however, this can be quite foul—but necessary. You will feel great after the first week.

Liver Cleanse

After the Epsom salt cleanse, a liver cleanse is next. Since everything in the body must be processed through the liver, it takes quite a lot of the load in regards to pollutants and toxins being eliminated from the system. There are many different methods to cleanse your liver naturally. You can do some research and choose one that feels right for you. Check more than one source and you will see a common thread emerge as to which foods are the best choice. I suggest the one that uses olive oil, grated beet, or fresh beet juice, with grated apple or fresh apple juice. Add a little lemon and you are set. Drink this before breakfast each day for two weeks. Many of the foods that I list in the upcoming pages are great support for your liver. Turmeric, lemon, garlic, walnuts, kale, and Brussels sprouts are just a few that are detoxifying for the liver. A healthy liver will make a huge difference in how much energy you feel.

Household Cleaning Supplies

It is also important to change all of your household cleansers to environmentally friendly products that will not pollute your home, body or air. I replaced all of my bathroom cleansers, dish detergent, laundry detergent, window cleaners, etc. All such products need to be in harmony with your body. There are many companies supplying very good cleaners, and I did not notice any lessening of cleaning ability when switching to body-friendly brands.

Body Cleansing Products

You have to do the same thing with anything you use to clean your body. I changed shampoo and conditioner to brands that were vegan based, sulphate and paraben free. Toothpaste should be all natural with no fluorides. Soap should be olive oil, or glycerin with all natural florals and herbals to scent. Any makeup, lip balms, body creams should be all natural as well. Coconut oil is a great body lotion. I buy organic whenever possible.

Body Brushing

This practice is very beneficial to removing toxins from the body. You take a cotton cloth and immerse it in hot water and ring it out and vigorously brush your entire body. This improves circulation quite dramatically and gets rid of adipose tissue, releasing toxins. Adipose tissue is body fat, and its main role is to store energy and insulate the body. Adipose tissue can affect other organ systems within the body that can lead to disease.

I still body brush almost every day, but I do not always use a hot cloth these days, I just use a dry cotton face cloth to stimulate my body before having a shower. The hot cloth should be used in the beginning for the maximum benefit.

Chapter 3.
MACROBIOTIC DIET

The most documented and successful diet for serious chronic illness of any sort—and especially cancer—is the macrobiotic diet. This is quite a strict form of eating, but if you are diligent, you will be amazed at the health benefits it yields. I started on this while I was in the Philippines and received a tailored-made diet, compiled for me by a man named Patrick Hamouy who cured himself of liver and intestinal cancer through a macrobiotic diet. You can contact him for your own personal consultation by going to patrick@therapies.com. Patrick is one of the best at this, and can personalize your diet to your specific illness. There are plenty of sites on the internet covering macrobiotics.

For breast cancer, Patrick tailored my diet to starve my body of any of the foods that would feed the cancer. So as a result, sugar and protein were my worst enemies. So even within the macrobiotic diet, I was restricted as to how much fruit and protein I was allowed. This increased my odds of success dramatically. I was allowed no sugars, only a bit of brown rice syrup occasionally. My protein was also limited to ten percent of the daily intake of food. This was in effect for six months. After the six months, I was allowed to increase the amount of natural fruit sugars and protein.

I have marveled at how my body loves this way of eating. I will not candy coat it, it's hard! I started while I was in the Philippines, where the only allowable items available to eat were white rice and steamed vegetables. I ate this for two solid weeks, three times a day, until I returned home to Canada. Let me tell you, it got old quickly. So when I finally arrived home and could have brown rice, oatmeal, barley, roasted vegetables, well I can tell you, it was like eating heaven sent food. Oatmeal never tasted so good before. A piece of fruit was like candy to me. As I followed this diet—and I did—very strictly, I noticed how satiated I felt after each meal, and how consistent my energy levels were. Before eating this way, I would often have a tired spell in the middle of the afternoon. Now I have unlimited energy. I never need to nap during the day, and I sleep great at night.

Now, three years into my macrobiotic diet, I have managed to make it my own. I love to eat. I have created many recipes that even people who have never eaten macrobiotic food enjoy. One of the purposes of this book is to share the wealth of my discoveries around creating tasty healthy macrobiotic dishes. I wish I had someone give me this sort of leg up at the beginning of my journey. You can find macrobiotic recipes on my blog page. There are also other recipes that I developed for eating when the cancer left my body, and I was able to move into a more expanded list of foods.

The basics of macrobiotic eating are listed below, and most of it comes from the information provided to me by Patrick Hamouy.

Protein is for growth and repairs. Carbohydrates are for energy. Vegetable protein is easier for the body to utilize than animal protein and is better for health and vitality. The human digestive system is 30 feet long (10 meters) and suitable for digesting plant material rather than animal protein. Animal and dairy proteins leave by-products such as cholesterol and fatty deposits when they are digested. These fatty deposits create the foundation for future illness to develop. Red meat, poultry and dairy products provide saturated fats that are harmful to our health. The recent change to a diet high in animal and dairy protein (such as the popular Atkins Diet) is responsible for many modern health problems and this includes increases in cancer, heart disease, diabetes and the break down of the immune system.

A combination of unrefined cereal grains and vegetables provide the basis for balanced nutrition. Cereal grains and vegetables, eaten together at the same meal, complement each other to form complete and balanced nutrition, which minimizes our need for animal proteins. White fish meat is better than poultry and other meats as it provides mainly unsaturated fats. Also unrefined cereal grains provide smooth and long-lasting energy. Animal and dairy foods lack carbohydrates, our main source of energy. They create cravings for refined carbohydrates and sugar. Refined grains such as potatoes and sugar give quick but short lasting energy. They also make our blood more acidic and rob our body of valuable nutrients in the digestive process. Unrefined cereal grains are digested and absorbed slowly into the body and create a more alkaline blood—when chewed slowly—which is the basis for better health and vitality. Their slow and even digestion provides enduring energy that is there when we need it.

Create variety in your cooking by selecting foods from different categories such as grains, soups, miso, beans, vegetables, allowable condiments, pickles and mix it up with an occasional food that you do not have on a regular basis. Cut your vegetables in different ways. Don't overcook vegetables. Adjust your cooking to incorporate foods during the different seasons.

Keep your food fresh. Never eat anything after three days. The energy of it has diminished greatly by then. Always cook fresh daily if possible, but it's okay to have leftovers for a couple of days. Take things out of the fridge and allow them to come to room temperature before eating them.

Use a variety of cooking methods. Pressure cooking is the ideal and preferred way to cook all rice. Boiling, blanching, steaming is all great as well. Oil sautéing, water sautéing, and stewing are good. Only occasionally should you grill, or deep fry; and coconut oil is the best for either of these as it produces no free radicals.

Traditionally, fifty percent of your diet is made up of grains, which can include barley, pearl barley, millet, corn, (corn on the cob), whole oats, rye, buckwheat, and quinoa. This also includes brown rice, both short and long grained. Occasional use grains are sweet brown rice, cracked wheat, couscous, bulgur, corn meal, (polenta) etc.

Vegetables should make up forty percent of your diet. This includes miso soup eaten each day, at least once or twice. Miso is a soybean and/or brown rice/barley paste. I found adding greens to my miso very delicious, especially seaweeds, as I am not a great lover of sea vegetables. Sea vegetables are different types of seaweeds that are used as vegetables. Some examples are dulse, nori, kombu, and wakame. There are unprocessed algae that are high in minerals. I also added chopped green onions, and a teaspoon of Bragg soy sauce to the mixture. Miso is a great fermented food that is key in the macrobiotic diet. It is teeming with natural probiotics that keep your intestinal track very healthy. Brine pickles are also a great natural probiotic food. Make sure they have been aged naturally in only sea salt, or make your own. Finally, ten percent of your diet should include proteins from beans, or bean products, nuts, tofu, and sea vegetables or fish.

A list of vegetables that are best for regular use (daily) are as follows:	Vegetables for occasional use (couple of times a week) are as follows:	Vegetables for infrequent use (once a week) are as follows:
leafy greens	celery	artichoke
bok choy	chives	aubergine
carrot tops	cucumber	asparagus
chinese cabbage	iceberg lettuce	avocado
daikon radish greens	green peas	bamboo shoots
dandelion greens	green beans	beets
kale	mushroom	fennel
leeks	squash	ferns
parsley	romaine lettuce	ginseng
spring cabbage	snap beans	okra
spring greens	snow peas	rhubarb
spring onions	and sprouts	spinach

turnip greens		sweet potato
watercress		swiss chard
broccoli		yams
brussels sprouts		
butternut squash		
cabbage		
cauliflower		
pumpkin		
onion		
red cabbage		
turnip		
shiitake mushrooms		
parsnips		
burdock		
carrots		
daikon radish		
dandelion root		
red radish		
white radish		

Bean choices for regular use include azuki beans, black soy beans, green or brown lentils. Occasional use are black eyed peas, kidney beans, lima beans, mung beans, chick peas or garbanzo beans, navy beans, pinto beans, soy beans, split peas or whole dried peas. Again, these should comprise no more than ten percent of your diet in the first six months.

Nuts and seeds are to be used occasionally, typically about a cup a week. These include pumpkin seeds, sesame seeds, almonds, chestnuts, hazelnuts, peanuts, walnuts and pecans. Avoid tropical nuts such as brazil, cashews, macadamia, and pistachio. Nut butters can also be used but more infrequently.

Occasional use of fruit is also allowed in the first six months, you can increase it after that time period. These include blueberries, blackberries, cantaloupe, raspberries, strawberries, watermelon, apples, apricots, cherries, grapes, peaches, plums and raisins. Citrus fruits such as oranges and limes are to be avoided as well as all tropical fruits and dried tropical fruits, which include banana, dates, figs, mango, papaya, and pineapple.

In conclusion, I would like to again stress some of the overarching philosophy around macrobiotic eating.

- One should eat organically grown food whenever possible.
- Avoid any GMOs (genetically modified foods).
- Whole grains should be used instead of refined grains.
- Always chew your food slowly and thoroughly.
- Sourdough bread is best. (Must use a natural sourdough starter)
- Fresh vegetables should be eaten at lunch and dinner.
- Use unrefined sea salt.
- Use unrefined oils such as sesame, olive, safflower, sunflower or corn instead of butter/fats.
- Brown rice syrup and barley malt should be used instead of sugar.
- Fish instead of chicken or meat.
- Proteins such as beans, tofu, seitan and tempeh instead of meat and cheese.
- Avoid ordinary teas and coffees. Drink organic herbal teas. Do not drink cold or iced beverages. This contributes to cysts.
- Choose cleaning materials from natural companies such as E-Cover. Avoid fluoride toothpaste, synthetically produced cosmetics, perfumes and any other harmful chemicals used in or on your body or around your personal environment.
- It is beneficial to wear cotton or linen next to your skin.
- Avoid using microwaves and non-stick cookware.
- Avoid sugar. This includes honey, maple syrup, agave, molasses, and corn syrup. Also avoid sugar substitutes such as aspartame, NutraSweet, saccharine, sorbitol, etc.
- Avoid deadly nightshade foods such as potatoes, red and green peppers, tomatoes, and pepper.
- Avoid processed foods, canned food, and commercial frozen foods.

- Avoid foods containing additives, coloring, flavoring, emulsifiers, and stabilizers.
- Avoid dairy.
- Create adequate ventilation in your home by regularly opening doors and windows rear round.
- Try to keep your home clean and orderly.
- Keep a significant number of green plants in rooms where you spend most of your time, including the bedroom.
- Sing a happy song each day.
- Try to take a half hour walk every day, regardless of the weather.
- Try cultivating a positive and bright mental outlook. Try to develop the mentality that can turn difficulties into challenges and adventures.
- Try to develop a deep sense of marvel and appreciation for all of life.
- Review and adjust your macrobiotic practice often.

While I have included what I feel are the primary aspects of the macrobiotic way of living and eating, you can certainly find more expanded lists of food and recipes on the internet, and I encourage you to read more sources on this way of eating. I highly recommend it, and I believe you will be very happy with your body from this way of eating not only as a way to rid your body of disease, but as a way of everyday living that gives you a great amount of joy and energy. It is important not to become too stressed around eating properly. Macrobiotic eating is a great tool to move you in the direction of a balanced healthy body. But the important word here is *balanced*. I was very strict in following this diet for the first year. I knew macrobiotic eating would give me a tremendous boost in ridding myself of the cancer, and my motivation was a desire to live and stay on the planet. When the body is in a state of low vibration or low frequency, it can manifest disease. Science is now starting to understand what sages through the ages have intuitively known. That everything is energy. Therefore, the higher your energy vibrates, the better the health of your body will be. This can be measured by megahertz. At the normal healthy level a human vibrates at a range of 62–68 hertz. At this level most people have very few ailments. People with cancer typically show a vibration of around 42 hertz.

The use of dietary changes and the consuming of higher vibrational foods is a great help in moving the body into a state of wellness. You cannot go instantly into a state of high vibration, it must be done incrementally. Eating foods that have a fresher higher energy is a tool to move you into a new state of being. If a person was continuously vibrating at a very high level, it would not matter what they ate. Disease cannot manifest in a body that has a high vibration. The macrobiotic diet is a step in a journey towards increasing your frequency. As I moved into a more healthy state of being, I realized that it was okay to eat foods that would be considered *unhealthy* from the macrobiotic perspective. I still use this way of eating as a guideline for the majority of my meals. So three years later, I follow the macrobiotic way of eating about eighty percent of the time, and I occasionally eat foods from the restricted list, such as chocolate, cheese, peppers, potatoes, etc., when I am out with friends, or sometimes I prepare them at home. I have learned to prepare them in the healthiest way possible and take great joy in eating these *treats*. All is a state of mind, so if you do decide to eat something that is not considered the highest energy choice, do not be fearful because of this choice. The most important thing you can do is enjoy it! We are here to take pleasure in life.

Chapter 4.
ACID FOODS VERSUS ALKALINE FOODS

There is a simple way for people to understand, biologically, how the body gets into a state of disease. When an acid situation prevails in the body, the body is actually receiving the message to decompose. This 'acidosis' is an increased acidity in the blood and other body tissues. One of the symptoms of acidosis is when oxygen and calcium are lacking. This acidic state sends out the message that the body is dying, and so the biology of the body responds accordingly. An *alkaline* state is the opposite of an *acidic* state, and many researchers say that cancer cannot live in an alkaline state. So it is very simple. When you choose foods that have less acidity, and are more of an alkaline composition, then you are giving your body a message of health and balance. I will state, yet again, that *balance* is the key. All great eating regimes, whether it is the Japanese macrobiotic diet or the Indian Ayurvedic diet, are based on the idea of yin versus yang or the optimum achievable balance. Three years later, I have incorporated the best of these two styles of eating for my own personal enjoyment. You can quickly check online what foods are acid based and which are more alkaline based.

Kale is an excellent alkaline-based food. Kale is full of calcium and is well known for its cancer fighting properties. The reason I named this book *Wake Up and Eat the Kale* is due to the resistance I often get from people when I tell them to eat kale. It can have a bit of a bitter taste at times, and is not the tastiest of all greens, however, its quality and quantity of nutrients goes unsurpassed in my opinion, and my great determination to heal myself overrode any lingering thoughts of not including it in my regular diet. I now love kale in all the ways I prepare it. I eat it raw; I make a tasty soup with it and also bake kale chips. They are surprisingly delicious.

Fermented Foods/Probiotics

The macrobiotic diet first introduced me to the beautiful benefits of fermented foods. This is a lost practice in today's fast food climate, but fermented foods were a staple in the diet of people throughout history.

Fermented foods are a great source of *good* bacteria. This beneficial bacteria is key to a balanced healthy ecosystem within the body and helps eat the *bad* bacteria, such as yeast, which most people have an over abundance of in their bodies today.

The most important and easily obtained fermented foods are naturally fermented sauerkraut and miso. Any vegetable can be naturally fermented by putting it in a glass jar with sea salt and water, allowing it to ferment at room temperature for about three days, then transferring it to the fridge. Miso can be bought at most health food stores; you will want one that is kept in the fridge and made from barley, rice and or soy. Miso is full of abundant live cultures and is quite an easy and tasty soup to make. I add green onions and some shredded sea vegetables, such as dulse, with mine.

Sourdough bread that is baked with only a natural sourdough starter is also a great fermented food. I eat sourdough bread on a regular basis.

Naturally fermented foods balance your intestines with their probiotic rich infiltration, and they also help your body to absorb nutrients more beneficially. They are a great addition to a diet that brings balance and harmony to the body.

Chapter 5.
RECIPES FOR THE BEGINNER

I decided to add some basic recipes for those of you who just want to get started on a cleansing diet and do not know where to begin. Macrobiotic eating can be a bit grim at first. It is quite a change, and I have developed many recipes over the past three years that I find fits with the detoxification of the body, but also are quite tasty.

I will be putting recipes on my blog page that are more comprehensive than the few listed here. As I healed, my diet changed and evolved. As a result, the selection and recipes I developed became quite extensive.

I love to cook, and I love to eat. In cooking, like so many endeavors, necessity is the mother of invention. To help people get started, I have included some basic recipes that I used at the beginning of the dietary part of my journey.

Breakfast

Oatmeal

- 1/2 cup of oatmeal
- 1 cup of water
- 1/2 tsp cinnamon

- 1/2 tsp sea salt
- 1/2 cup of almond or coconut milk
- 1 small apple peeled and diced
- 1/2 cup of fresh blueberries

Put the oatmeal, water, cinnamon and salt into a saucepan and bring to a boil. Cook until desired consistency and take off of burner. Stir in the milk, apple, and blueberries. Serve warm.

Breakfast Smoothie

- 1 cup of berries/fruit
- 2 cups of liquid. (Combination of unsweetened coconut milk, almond milk and water)
- 1 tbsp of almond butter
- 2 tbsp of ground flax
- 2 tbsp of chia seed
- 2 cups of diced kale and or spinach

Put all ingredients in a food processor or handheld processor and pulse until smooth. Add or subtract liquid as desired. This will up your level of fiber and antioxidants.

Buckwheat Apple Pancakes

Prepare apples by roasting them first.

- 3 apples peeled and diced. Granny Smith and Macintosh are great.
- 1 tsp cinnamon
- Juice of 1/2 lemon

Preheat oven to 400°F. Combine apples, cinnamon and lemon juice in a small bowl. Stir them and then place the mixture on a cookie sheet. Bake for 20 minutes and let stand for 10.

Pancake mixture
- 3/4 cups of buckwheat flour

- 1/2 tsp of cinnamon
- 1/4 tsp of sea salt
- 1 cup of blueberries
- 3 tbsp unsweetened almond milk
- 3 tbsp water
- 2 tbsp sunflower oil
- 1/2 tsp vanilla extract
- 1 flax egg substitute (combine 1 tbsp of ground flax-seed with 3 tbsp water and let sit for 2 minutes.)

Stir the flour and cinnamon and salt in a bowl. Add blueberries and stir. Combine the milk, water, and one tablespoon of the sunflower oil and vanilla in a separate bowl. Stir the flax substitute into the milk mixture. Pour the milk mixture into the flour bowl, mixing just until combined, using a whisk. If the batter is too thick or stiff, add a little more milk. Heat the remaining tablespoon of oil in a pan or griddle over medium low heat and then spoon mixture onto the oil. Buckwheat flour browns quickly, so make sure the pan is not too hot. Once the edges are slightly browned and a few bubbles appear, flip the pancakes over. Top with roasted apples.

Sourdough Bread Toast/Sandwiches

I love to have a toasted sandwich from time to time, and so this is great for breakfast, lunch or supper.

- Sourdough Bread (from a baker that uses a natural starter, not yeast!)
- oil drizzled over bread or toast
- green onions
- garlic salt
- greens, lettuce, kale or spinach
- cucumber,
- organic mustard or mayo (use a brand that has no sugar)
- salt to taste

Cereal

I often have a big bowl of cereal combined with many of the ingredients I put in the smoothie.

- corn flakes or a combination any other cereal that has no sugar in it. Fruit juice sweetened is okay. diced apple, pear or fresh blueberries or any allowed fruit
- 2 tbsp chia seed
- 2 tbsp ground flax
- 1 tbsp sesame seeds
- 6 crumbled walnuts
- cinnamon to taste
- Almond milk or creamy coconut milk

Lunch

Squash Soup

- 2 tbsp extra virgin olive oil
- 2 small onions diced
- 3 garlic cloves minced
- 2 large carrots diced
- 2 celery stalks chopped
- 1 large butternut squash, peeled and diced
- 1 sweet potato diced
- 6 cups of water
- 1/2 cup of loosely packed fresh parsley
- 1/2 tsp each of ground bay leaf, thyme and turmeric
- 1 tbsp of fresh minced ginger root
- 1 tsp of sea salt
- Juice of half a lemon

Sauté the onions and garlic in the olive oil. Add all other ingredients and bring to a boil. Let simmer for about 40 minutes or until vegetables are tender. I like owning an immersion hand blender for pureeing soups, they make it so easy. Puree the soup until smooth, if you like your soup to be more robust and thick, add a tablespoon or two of brown rice flour to thicken. Also you can add more salt to taste.

Add a piece of bread with oil, and you have a healthy nutrient rich lunch.

Kale Soup

- 2 tbsp olive oil
- 3 large garlic cloves
- 2 medium onions
- 6 cups of shredded kale
- 6 cups of water
- 1 1/2 tsp sea salt
- 2 tsp turmeric
- 1 tbsp tahini or almond butter
- 3 tbsp brown rice flour

Sauté onions and garlic in olive oil, just until starting to brown. Shove as much kale as you can get into the pot, about 6 cups. It will cook down quickly. Add 6 cups of water and bring to a boil. Simmer for about 20 minutes. Take off burner and add tahini or almond butter, and flour and puree until smooth and green. This is surprisingly yummy and satisfying.

Salad

- Greens of any kind, spinach, lettuce, arugula, or kale
- Chopped apple, pear, or blueberries
- Chopped green onions
- Shredded beet or carrot or zucchini
- cut up celery or cucumber
- Add any nuts, seeds, or small amount of dried fruit such as raisins
- Top with crumbled corn chips or Mary's Seed Crackers

Homemade Salad Dressing
- 3/4 cup of sunflower or safflower oil

- 1/4 cup of juice from brine pickles, either home-made or naturally fermented sauerkraut
- 2 tbsp lemon juice
- 1 tbsp apple cider vinegar
- 1 tbsp prepared organic mustard
- 2 tbsp brown rice syrup
- 1 tbsp tahini
- 1 tbsp almond butter
- 1 tsp garlic salt or powder

Puree with hand held processor until rich and creamy. Store in fridge.

Supper

Miso with Seaweed

Prepare Miso as directed

Add chopped seaweed and green onions to the mixture and let stand for a few minutes and serve.

I had this every day for my first year to enrich my system with abundant cultures and nutrients from the sea vegetables.

Brown rice with Roasted Vegetables

Prepare Brown Rice

Roasted Vegetables:

Use broccoli, carrots, onions, beets, mushrooms, cauliflower, etc. Cut up a combination of desired vegetables and put in a glass ovenproof container. Drizzle with olive oil and shake garlic salt and regular salt over the mixture. Bake at 400°F for 40 to 45 minutes, uncovered, until vegetables are roasted but not burnt.

Add some olive oil to the rice and mix, serving the vegetables over the rice. This is much like a stir fry but with a more satisfying flavor.

Brown Rice Pasta with Mushrooms

Cook a small bag of brown rice pasta as directed. Remember to take it off the heat when it is still *al dente* (that means a bit firm) and always use olive oil in the boiling water and rinse it after it is cooked. It takes a little practice to cook brown rice pasta to a satisfying consistency, but you will get the hang of it.

Sauté 3 cloves of garlic, 2 small onions and 8 large mushrooms in a frying pan in 2 tablespoons of olive oil until they are slightly browned. Add this mixture to the drained pasta. Add 3 tablespoons of Bragg Soya Sauce and a quarter cup of olive oil and stir. Serve hot. This tastes like a meaty dish due to the mushrooms.

Hearty Vegetarian Stew

- 2 tbsp sunflower oil
- 3 garlic cloves minced
- 2 tbsp minced fresh ginger
- 1/4 tsp each of allspice and ground coriander
- 1/2 tsp each of turmeric, cinnamon, and cumin
- l large sweet potato diced
- 1 medium zucchini diced
- 2 carrots washed and diced
- 1/2 head of a small cabbage diced or shredded
- 2 small turnips diced
- 1/4 head of cauliflower diced
- 1 9 oz can of chickpeas, drained and rinsed
- 1/2 cup of fresh cilantro

Sauté in oil the garlic, ginger, spices and coriander until slightly browned. Add all the vegetables. Pour in enough water to cover the vegetables and cook covered for about 25 to 30 minutes. Just until the veggies are tender but not overcooked. Take our about a third of the mixture and puree it until thick and then add back into the stew. Mix in the chickpeas with the salt and simmer on low for about 10 minutes. Add in the cilantro and serve over brown rice.

Snacks

Kale Chips

These are quite crispy and tasty. They can replace a potato chip.
- 1 bunch of kale
- 1 tbsp olive oil
- sesame seeds
- apple cider vinegar (optional)

Preheat the oven to 375°F. Remove the stems from the kale, and wash and dry the leaves. Tear them into bite size pieces. Rub each piece with a bit of olive oil, it will feel much like rubbing a soft leather. They will be supple but not oily. It sinks in quite easily. Line a cookie sheet with parchment paper and place the kale leaves on top. Sprinkle a couple of teaspoons of sesame seeds, and then you can also spray/flick with your fingertips some apple cider vinegar over them as well. Finish off with a very light dash of salt, as it does not take much salt to make these chips taste salty. Bake 10–15 minutes until the edges are brown but not burnt.

Popcorn

Organic popcorn is another tasty snack. Cook on the stove with an organic sunflower oil, and lightly salt.

Naturally fermented Sauerkraut/Pickles

Another great addition to your diet is naturally fermented pickles or sauerkraut. I buy a brand called Bubbies that is quite delicious. But you can also make your own.

Brine Pickles

Boil 3 cups of water and 1 tsp of salt. Let cool. Place a 3-inch piece of kombu and slices of carrot, onion, daikon radish, broccoli, cauliflower etc. in a jar with the cooled salt water. All vegetables should be immersed in the water. Cover with cheese cloth. Keep in a cool dark place for 2 to 3 days and then refrigerate. Serve in 3 to 5 days. This is full of good bacteria and great for the intestinal tract.

Chapter 6.
SUPPLEMENTS

In conjunction with my new diet, I still opted to take supplements, as I felt I might not get the concentration of greens (which offer the most alkaline properties) that I needed from just eating the food. There is a great healing modality called the Gerson Diet, and you can research this as well, it is quite interesting and has had very successful results for many people. However, I did not use the Gerson Diet as it uses a lot of fruit juicing and this would not be conducive with the sugar-free diet I was following to treat my breast cancer. I did feel their use of green drinks to be quite a sound practice, as it involves keeping the body in an alkaline state, which inhibits the growth of cancer. So together with my naturopath we came up with a list of supplements that would help me further support my body. The list included vitamin C 6000 mg/day for the first year, selenium, astragalus, calcium magnesium, beta carotene, vitamin D, green supplements such as phytogreens, chlorella , and spirulina along with coenzyme Q10 and a supplement called I3C, known as Indole-3-carbinol. This is a supplement that is made from concentrated cruciferous vegetables such as cabbage, kale, broccoli, bok choy, and various other greens that are known for their anti-cancer properties. However, it is produced in a concentrated form and is considered a natural alternative to the drug tamoxifen. There have been many clinical trials using I3C showing conclusively its effectiveness in treating breast and other cancers.

In addition to supplements, the following are other practices I felt would aid me in keeping a healthy inner environment and facilitate my body's ability to rid itself of the cancer.

Apple Cider Vinegar

Apple cider vinegar is a great addition to anyone's health regime. It is the first thing naturopathic doctors start people on to help them get their bodies in a state of balance. It helps move the body into a more alkaline state and is great for killing off yeast. A tablespoon in three liters of water is the daily prescription and should be taken for a month. Then you can intermittently dose yourself as needed. Great for stomach discomfort as well. Choose an organic variety with the so-called *mother* included. Apple cider vinegar in its natural state means that the mother is intact. This ball of living enzymes is packed full of goodness and is mostly responsible for the beneficial properties of the vinegar. You can enhance the mother by leaving the bottle in sunlight every so often.

Apple cider vinegar is a great liver cleanser as well. It should be used periodically as one recovers throughout the continuation of life.

Turmeric

I take half a teaspoon in water twice a day. I did this for the first year, and as I moved into the second year, I did it every second day. This information about the absolute value of turmeric came to me well before I was ever diagnosed.

I heard the author of a book called *Foods That Fight Cancer* on a radio show one afternoon, and I found it fascinating when he described his creation of new chemotherapy drugs in his biochemical laboratory came from his observations and studies of plants in their natural environment. He stated that, if he had to pick the most important food that would benefit people, with cancer it would be turmeric. It creates a most inhospitable environment for cancer in the body. You can read more about this by going to his site at www.richardbeliveau.org.

Naturopathic doctors also recommend turmeric to people dealing with cancer. An interesting side effect of ingesting turmeric on a regular basis is that it gives you a lovely natural looking tan. I noticed after the first year that people during the winter months would always ask me where I had been down south because I looked so tanned. Turmeric is an active ingredient in self-tanning lotions, but it is much more natural and beneficial to ingest it.

Asparagus

A friend of my brother had heard very good things around the healing properties of asparagus, and I always listen when the universe sends me messages. So I tried the asparagus for about one month. I think it helps to switch it up with different healing foods. So I took four tablespoon of pureed asparagus morning and evening.

Lemon Grass Tea

My husband was told about three times in one week about people who had experienced great success with cancer from drinking lemon grass tea. It comes from Israel, and there is quite a write up on the internet from many people claiming the amazing healing properties with cancer from this tea. So again, I drink it quite often, and take a break every once in a while and then go back to it. It has a very refreshing pleasant taste. I feel very good drinking it.

Fresh Lemon

During the second year, I started alternating between turmeric and lemon. So every second day I would squeeze fresh organic lemon into a cup of warm water and drink it first thing in the morning about a half hour before breakfast. Fresh lemon in warm water is a great liver detoxifier as well as a known anti-cancer fruit.

Castor Oil

Castor oil is used by naturopathic doctors for inflammation. So I was advised to put it on my breast and liver and allow it to soak in over a period of time. I usually did this at night before going to bed. It is important to note that no heat should be used as you do not want to have increased blood flow to either area.

Siberian Pine Nut Oil

I came across this amazing healing remedy while reading the book *Anastasia* from the Ringing Cedars series. This is a phenomenal series about a woman in the wilds of Russia who lives all by herself with her two grandfathers, aged ninety-six and one hundred and twenty respectively—these remarkable people live a pure life surrounded by nature and connected to the cosmic grid of the universe. They are in touch with nature to the highest degree and can communicate with animals and live totally off of what nature provides. This fascinating true story is about a Russian businessman who meets with this beautiful young woman who changes his life and the lives of millions of people worldwide through their co-creation and intention. From this special place in Russia comes a cedar oil that has miraculous healing qualities, and is now made available to people all over the world. You can read about this story and the oil by going to www.ringingcedarsofrussia.com. I have used this oil on two different occasions, about a year apart, and feel that it was very beneficial to my body. It has anti-aging properties as well, and I did notice that, both times I was taking it, people remarked that I had a glow that seemed to emanate from me.

Essiac

I used Essiac in tincture form for the first year, one teaspoon in the morning and one teaspoon before bed. I then started brewing my own Essiac tea, as it was much cheaper, and I decided that I could do without the alcohol in the tincture. I had read an article on Essiac in my early twenties, and like many other singular events in my life that made no sense at the time, I knew intuitively that I would use it some day, so had programmed myself to remember its name in case I ever needed it.

I only read the amazing story of Rene Caisse recently, and was surprised to find I had another connection as to why Essiac resonated with me. This amazing woman was a nurse in the 1920s, and in her work met a woman who had breast cancer, but had no resources to have surgery. She was given a herbal concoction from a native aboriginal friend and it cured her. This woman gave the recipe to Rene Caisse, and she brewed it up and tried it on a couple of relatives who had cancer and cured them both. So she started offering Essiac for free from a clinic that she opened for three hours a day. Needless to say, the authorities got involved, many doctors wanted to shut her down, but some thought she was doing good work. One of the doctors who supported her was Sir Frederick Banting, who was a relative of mine on my father's side. Banting offered her his facility to do research on this promising cancer remedy. He found benefits from this herbal decoction to have great benefits for the pancreas, and many people today use Essiac to help control their diabetes. Sir Frederick Banting was also working on a cure for cancer at the time of his death. You can read more about this story by going to www.healthfreedom. info/Cancer%20Essiac.htm.

Essiac is considered a blood purifier, and I alternately use a few others just to mix it up. Here are the recipes.

Essiac (This is a decoction as opposed to the tea variety which are considered infusions).

- 1 lb. burdock root
- 1 lb. sheep sorrel (roots included, very important) powdered
- 4 oz. turkey rhubarb powdered
- 4 oz. slippery elm powdered

Combine all ingredients together and then put one ounce of herbs into a covered pot with thirty-two ounces of water. Bring to a boil and let simmer for 10 minutes. Leave overnight covered. In morning, bring to a boil once again, then strain into a sterilized glass jar, and refrigerate. Drink four ounces at room temperature twice a day.

While I include the recipe for Essiac here for those who would like to brew their own, it is very difficult to get sheep sorrel root. All of the

Essiac available for sale today in health food stores does not include the root, just the leaves. The original recipe states that the root is a very important part of the remedy, so it was serendipitous for me to find that it grows in abundance in my neck of the woods. I have a gardener friend who gathers it for me regularly, and I have a large supply of it dried, and so have taken to making my own, and as a result many people come to me in search of my brand. I wanted the purest formula I could manufacture. I am sure there are benefits to all forms of Essiac. The original form is of course the most desired, and therefore I am happy to offer it to those who want the purer form.

You can also switch it up with these other teas I found to be of great value in my healing.

Lymphatic Purifying Tea—Blood Purifying Tea

- 1 part echinacea
- 1 part astragalus
- 1 part cleavers
- 1 part goldenseal

Lymphatic Purifying Tea—Blood Purifying Tea

- 2 parts burdock root
- 2 parts comfrey
- 1 part peppermint
- 1 part wormwood/1 part nettle

Daikon Radish Tea

You can steep dried daikon radish in hot water for about ten minutes to make a very strong tea that has great benefits for the body. In the early days, I also grated up a quarter cup each of fresh daikon radish and carrot and brought them to a boil for a few minutes in water and then consumed it as a soup. This is a macrobiotic treatment for ridding the body of little tumors.

Most health food stores will have these herbal tea products available in their bulk sections.

Water

It is extremely beneficial to drink at least two liters of water each day. In the beginning, three is even better. Hydration and the efficient removal of toxins in the body is very important. Water is what we are mostly made up of. Choose water that is clean, with as few impurities as you can manage. Spring water is best. You do not want fluoride or chlorine in your water. The purer the water, the better. Your goal is to have *live* water in your system. Most water is dead water due to the manipulation it has gone through especially in cities with water treatment systems. One is better off with well water, or finding a place to get natural spring water. I am lucky that I live on a lake with a pristine water source. During the majority of the year, I take my water directly from the lake. I take it from a depth of three feet from the surface water, in a clear glass bottle, and let it sit in the sun for three hours so as to let the ultraviolet rays purify it. This also allows me to have the abundant nutrients that accompany natural water from the earthy vegetation flowing into the lake. Of course, not everyone has access to natural water, so just do the best you can.

There is a very interesting man in Japan named Masaru Emoto. He revolutionized our understanding of water, using a highly unusual method of observation. He froze water crystals with the expectation that they should look like snow crystals. In the course of playing with this concept, he found that tap water and distilled water had no beautiful crystals. They were disfigured. He found that water taken from pristine lakes and rivers had beautifully formed crystals. He further experimented and noticed that the distilled water when he spoke kind words to it—or played good music or prayed to it—would develop beautiful crystals. He found the water would have disfigured crystals if he did the opposite to this. You can view more about this man and his process by visiting his site at www.masaru-emoto.net.

This concept was evidenced to me again by my sister-in-law, who created her own experiment around this idea as a school project with her daughter to show her the effects of the vibration of love. She cooked up a pot of white rice, and divided the contents into two sterilized mason jars. On one of the jars she labeled the word love, and the other jar was labeled with the word hate. Every day they would pick up the love jar and give it their loving thoughts, sometimes dancing with it in joyful intention. Alternatively, because they felt they could not actually hate the other jar, they just ignored it. Three months later—I kid you not—the love jar still had perfectly white rice, while the hate jar had brownish black ooze inside it, covered in mold. I saw this in person when I visited them, and I even asked them to send it to me on Facebook, a month after I had initially seen it, and still the love jar was white. This post was shared many times by people on Facebook because of the visual impact of this experiment.

Since every person gives off a magnetic field, or energy field, your thoughts and intentions can actually be measured. There are interesting studies around this. As was done with the water, you can do the same thing with food, as evidenced by the above rice experiment. Altering the energy of your food works the same as the changing of the water crystals with the loving intent etc. I always give an energetic thought to whatever goes into my body, whether it be appreciation for a delicious meal I am about to eat, or a purifying intention around a food or beverage that I feel is not as fresh or of the highest vibration. I add my intent to raise the vibration of the food. This is not unlike the historical blessing of food in religious cultures. All is energy and your intention can alter the frequency of it.

Chapter 7.
USING A NATUROPATHIC DOCTOR

My family started seeing a naturopathic doctor a few years prior to my developing cancer. This was mostly in response to my husband's acid reflux, and he had remarkable results with the naturopathic doctor's remedies after traditional medicine failed to affect a cure for this health crisis he was enduring. He was miserable for about five years before seeing the naturopath. His stomach was raw and hurt continuously due to the inflammation and drugs he was taking. He once went on a brown rice diet for two solid weeks, just so he could feel better. A brutal endeavor I can tell you. He was quite grumpy during those two weeks, but his stomach did feel better. However, this sort of drastic remedy is not a pleasant way to live and could not realistically be sustained indefinitely. We finally tried a naturopathic doctor and he had complete success in getting his acid reflux under control during that time. As a result of this experience, I became a great advocate of seeing naturopathic doctors, as they are trained to deal with healing the entire body, and bringing it into balance. They are also educated in the understanding of pharmaceutical drugs and the effects on the body in combination with natural healing supplements. I used to have chronic urinary tract infections from the young age of nine until I was in my late forties. After seeing the naturopath and having the Carroll Food Test, I found that I was intoler-ant to cane sugar and potato. As a result of a lifetime of eating these foods, this intolerance kept my body in a state of irritation which manifested in my body as bladder infections. After taking these foods out of my diet, my bladder problems went away. I am suggesting that many people may find a balanced way forward with the overall health of their body and their lifestyle by finding a naturopathic doctor that you feel comfortable with and using them appropriately for general maintenance of the body or for health issues that can be greatly helped by a natural approach.

I will stress here, again, that anyone who is undergoing chemotherapy, radiation, surgery, or any other illness that involves the use of medically prescribed drugs, will absolutely need to see a naturopathic doctor in conjunction with their regular doctor to be able to use many of my healing modalities—*especially* the use of homeopathic remedies, herbals and food supplements. These often contain high levels of certain vitamins and some of these can conflict with certain medications and be toxic in the system. Naturopathic doctors are perfectly trained to help facilitate the orchestration of this. I used Dr. Sarah Tanner, and you can view her site to gain more information on naturopathy by going to www.natural-choices.ca.

Chapter 8.
CHAKRAS

Chakras are the energy centers, or life force of the body. They are located inside the body. There are seven major chakras, and they govern our psychological properties.

If we were able to see the chakras—and many clairvoyants can—we would observe a colored wheel approximately the size of our fist continuously revolving or rotating. They begin at the base of the spine and finish at the top of the head. Each chakra vibrates at a different speed and has a corresponding color. You can go online and find many different sites that have great visual examples of the chakras, and how each color and chakra relates to different aspects of the psychological properties.

Blocked energy in any of these chakras can often lead to illness, so it is important to recognize the importance of these energy centers and to keep this energy flowing freely.

When the chakras are out of alignment, this will cause imbalance in the physical body. So understanding that everything is energy or life force will help you to want to bring your energy levels back to the optimum balance. This is done by being willing to deal with repressed emotions such as anger, shame, guilt, feelings of unworthiness etc. This is imperative to opening up your chakras so they can flow with ease.

You must commit to bringing painful unwanted parts of yourself to light. This can be deep and elusive, but you must persevere. There are many buried painful moments lying just under the surface of your everyday awareness, wanting to be brought up and released. The ability to allow this without judging yourself will clear your chakras of old stagnant energy that is clouding them. Sound and toning can also be a catalyst to bringing this stuff to the surface. I have done all of this and continue to work on the bits that can still come up from time to time. I did the lion's share of this exercise in the early days of my cancer, and it helped me greatly to heal. I expand on this concept many times throughout the book.

Chapter 9.

YOGA

Yoga is a Sanskrit word for the physical, mental and spiritual practices to attain permanent peace. The stilling of the changing states of the mind. Yoga has also been popularly defined as "union with the divine". Many studies have been done promoting the health benefits of doing yoga.

When I first started doing yoga on a regular basis, I went to a woman who had developed her own style of yoga based on her awareness of being able to actually see a person's energy field. I learned much from her about how everything is energy and vibration. Material items and events are just energy. Energy happens first, and the physical matter or event comes about as a result of the energetic thrust or intention that precedes it. So, understanding yoga can be very beneficial to unlocking repetitive or stagnant energy patterns that most of us are entrenched in, from the current life, and also past lives. The energetic body is created in dimensions higher than the third dimension and is not visible to the average naked eye, so our physical bodies become bogged down or out of alignment due to the amount of movement we engage in continuously. Trees for example hold their magnetic fields faithfully because they stay in one place. Therefore special practices such as yoga realign our physical forms, taking us out of an energetic slouch. If you watch cats, they hold yoga postures all day. They sleep in a very meditative way. Watch a cat or dog get up from a sleep, and the first thing they will do is a pose in yoga called the puppy dog stretch, and everyone has seen an animal do this pose. Doing yoga correctly patterns you with your light body, which regenerates your physical body. The rewards of correct alignment are health, joy, bliss, and a genuine appreciation for the flow of regeneration. Yoga has been popularized recently as a form of exercise, but it has far more reaching benefits than just exercise.

I experienced the tangible results of all this when I started doing yoga regularly. Some postures are simple and quite easy to do, and others are more challenging to hold in the correct postures. It is the moving into the correct postures, the ongoing attainment of perfecting the postures, that yields the energetic benefits. I heard my yoga instructor say many times that, if one holds the posture until they shake, or hold it continuously for three minutes, they will move the energy profoundly. I certainly did not achieve this in the first days, but with time I found I could hold the poses longer, and it became easier. At the end of a yoga session, you will feel the difference in how much better and more peaceful you feel. This I will guarantee. As important as the poses is the meditation that follows the end of a yoga class. Most styles of yoga end their class with a meditation or relaxation period. This is when all that you have done in class becomes integrated into the whole. A great feeling of peace and serenity is usually what one feels when they have completed a yoga class. It is important to be discerning in finding the right style of yoga or yoga instructor. Try a few different classes—the person who *feels right* will be the most comfortable for you. Yoga is a great practice to incorporate into your life. Don't worry about whether you are in the best shape or not to start, just begin where you are. It is beneficial for everyone.

Breathing

I cannot emphasize enough how important breathing is. There are people who have cured themselves of various illnesses just by breathing. Breath is life force—period! Most people breathe very shallowly, in and out of the chest area. You need to breathe deep into the lower belly. Long and slow breaths are best. The more often you do it, the better the results. There is a lot more to it than you would think. And the majority of people do not breathe properly. It was first brought to my attention by a friend of mine who practices reiki and is an all around amazing healer. When she first met me, she told me my eyes were very busy, always darting to and fro, and that I needed to be more peaceful. Then she told me to start breathing from my belly, big deep breaths. Once you start breathing deeply and often, you will wonder how you could have ever breathed any other way. I can always tell now when I am holding or resisting my breath. I start to feel stressed and anxious. Then I breathe in deeply and slowly and let it out the same way. A few of these and you feel great again. Being conscious of your breath also brings you into the present moment. So imagine the benefits if you breathed properly all day long.

I listened to a woman named Ellie Drake speak on a show called Blog Talk Radio about her dynamic success as an entrepreneur. She attributed her success solely to her understanding of successful breathing. I was fascinated to hear what she had to say. Apparently she started working for a telephone sales company and was wildly successful at selling. She associated her success to her intuitive ability to read people when she was speaking with them. She felt she could read them because she was more centered in her feminine power, as a result of breathing deep belly breaths, with the exhale coming out as a contented aahh sound. This is known as cleansing breath in yoga. She further discovered that such an exhale releases the love hormone oxytocin, and as a result, makes a person feel great. It also makes people more attracted to you. Men on the other hand release adrenaline, as they are designed to do. Women in the workplace in our modern times try to co-exist in the business world by competing with men on their terms, and as a result often release adrenaline and this leads to feelings of stress and anxiety. This woman discovered that, by staying in her feminine power with the belly breath, she was refreshed and very focused at all times. Those engaging with her could feel this and were more attracted and felt better around her. As a result she successfully runs seven businesses. She does state, though, that all new people being hired by her companies are informed of the regularity of hearing her make these deep moaning breaths at intermittent times during the day.

Many times in the early part of my healing I would wake up at night and feel very tense or stressed, and I would immediately take slow deep breaths. Very soon I would feel centered and peaceful and would easily fall back to sleep. I was educated much more about the health and spiritual benefits of breathing when I began doing yoga. I highly recommend taking a regular yoga class, and also becoming educated on the various breathing techniques that can help you immensely by bringing more life force or *prana* into your body. There are many great examples of breathing on YouTube.

Stretching

I learned the value of stretching when I started practicing yoga. Everyone has had moments where they have not felt at ease in their physical body. Since the body is really just energy, stretching kind of unsticks the uncomfortable feeling you can get in your body when you are not feeling well. I would often wake up in the middle of the night in the early days after the cancer diagnosis, and I could feel my body was tightened up, constricted. I just did not feel good. I would then stretch my entire body, twisting and turning, with arms raised above my head, and my feet reaching as far as they could. I would then take deep breaths right into the core of my belly and let them out with a great vocal release. I have to tell you, I felt wonderful after this. My body just let go. It released the energy that I was holding onto. I would then easily fall back to sleep. Often I would do this three or four times a night. Each time, the release would work beautifully. I also suggest lying on a mat any place on the floor—or on a bed—and practice letting your body move in ways it is not used to doing anymore. Like a baby, or small child. Watch how they take their feet and try to put them in their mouths, or the amazing ways they twist and turn while laying on their backs. They know no limitations and naturally move in a way that relaxes them; they intuitively know how to let energy move through their bodies. Let your body guide you to move in ways that you have not moved in a long time. Do not force any movement, just relax into whatever way your body wants to move, and let go. Enjoy. You will see the benefits of this when you try it.

Grounding/Earthing

Everything is energy at the micro level. If you were to see your physical body at the quantum level of existence, you would see a field of atoms spinning, with quite a lot of space in between them. All one needs do to effect healing is to change the pathways of energy in the body. All disease is a result of energy that is stagnant. You need to create higher vibrational energy in the body. All the things I have done and written about so far will affect the vibration of your body in a positive way if you choose to makes changes in your own mind and body. By changing existing patterns in your life, on any level, whether it is with food, or exercise, or by changing how you relate to yourself, to others, or to the world at large, you will create new energy pathways. This is the essence of living. Everything you experience is in a state of frequency or vibration, and disease exists in a state of low vibration, a stagnation of energy, whereas health and happiness are in a state of higher vibration, or the ease and flow of energy. This can be measured in megahertz.

Most people today get their energy from others. Have you ever noticed how interactions with some people leave you exhausted, while other people can make you feel peaceful and calm in their presence. The difference is the size of a person's energy field and at what rate they are vibrating. So, if a person is vibrating very high, you may find their presence soothing and pleasant—while another person who is vibrating at a lower rate may appear angry or tense and you will feel more stressed while in their company. One of the reasons why more disease exists in the world is because most people have lost their connection to the earth as a result of living in cities. Pavement covers the earth in the cities, therefore the quantity and quality of natural green space is very diminished within urban centers. People have lost their connection to the earth, and therefore have less energy available to them. Energy is also available from the air, yet the quality of that is very poor in most cities as well.

One of the best ways to enhance your energy and affect a more healthy state in the body is by being grounded. I am sure many of you have observed people meditating and chanting, "ohm." Most do not realize the huge benefit and significance of this practice. The vibration of the sound *ohm*, is the closest one can come to the actual vibration of the earth itself, and it brings one into a more harmonious state in the body. Just sit and ohm away for a while and you will feel the difference. Being in resonance with the earth itself makes a person feel more balanced. You can draw energy from the earth by being outside in nature, sitting on the ground, swimming in a lake or the ocean, and just by walking barefoot on the grass. A really great experience is to fully cover yourself in sand at the beach. Being encased in the sand right up to your head is very healing. The energy emanating from the earth is very pure. It is called *prana* in yoga, or *chi* in martial arts. Sit on the ground and let yourself become quiet, and allow the beautiful energy of the earth permeate your body and your soul. You will feel quite uplifted after doing this. Try to be out in nature for part of every day. In the summer, I swim in my lake at least once every day, and I feel quite energized and grounded each and every time. I made this part of my healing regime right from the very beginning.

Dr. James Oschman, who specializes in bio-physics and energy medicine, has quite a lot of information on this, and you can Google him to read more. The essence of his research is that walking barefoot on the earth heals people of disease by the transfer of free electrons which are antioxidants into the body from the earth.

Meditation

Meditation is a practice that allows one to regulate the internal musings of one's mind. A practice to achieve a state of empty mind and a feeling of peacefulness. To let go of thoughts. To go within. I could go on at great length about the practice and benefit of meditation. Is it beneficial? Absolutely. Is it easy? For some yes, and for some no. Personally, I am in the no category. I have never found it easy to mediate. I have, on occasion, been more successful at this than other times, to my great delight. Because when you actually are successful at achieving a state whereby your thoughts are not running the internal show, it is quite a beautiful experience. You do feel blissful, and content. Peaceful and accepting. However, it's often difficult to silence the ongoing chatter of the mind, and that is what most people find challenging when trying to meditate successfully. It takes a commitment to enter into productive meditation. You have to sit down and clear your mind often—and not judge yourself when nothing happens. Over time, you will find that it gets easier and you will have interesting things happen, and you will start to see the benefits of this practice.

Personally I find that meditation is much like acceptance, or surrender. I find I am most successful in reaching the exalted state when I just let go. Don't try. I take a few deep belly breaths and let them out noisily. I feel my body relaxing, and I tell myself that I don't have anywhere to go, I have nothing to do at this moment, and I just sink into my body, and allow it to be what it wants to be in that moment. Any thoughts that try to come up, I let them keep on going. I don't pay any attention to them. After a few minutes of this, you just seem to be in a state of suspended animation, almost trance or dreamlike, just being. Keep at it if you don't find it easy the first few times, you will come to enjoy and experience the profound levels of awareness and peacefulness that come from meditation.

As you become more adept and find it easier to meditate, you may then start having altered state experiences. You may start to notice that visual images will appear. My husband is great at this. He has only to shut his eyes and relax and all of a sudden it's like he has a movie going on behind his eyes. He often tells me of the interesting things he sees, most of it he can't make any sense of, he just observes the images and then lets them go. This is actually the opening of what is called the *third eye*, which is located energetically in the middle of your brow area. This is one of the seven chakras. The third eye is commonly portrayed symbolically as the Egyptian Eye of Horus. It is the eye that can see into the multiverse or into the dimensions that transcend third dimensional time and space. If this does not make any sense to you, it can be a bit disconcerting at first, and you will probably react by thinking about what you are seeing. This usually stops the process, as the altered state comes about when one is in a condition of total relaxation. Thinking about what you see will put you into a state of judging the experience—which will shut it down. It is always best to enjoy whatever is going on with no attachment to what you are seeing in the minds eye.

As well as visuals, you can have auditory experiences too. I often will hear someone say my name, quite loudly at times. It clearly is being heard from within though, not from an external source, and this too can be quite an interesting experience. Sometimes I see beautiful colors, all swirling around, with some being more pronounced than others. Symbols can often appear as well, ones that will make no sense to you, and others that you may recognize. Bright lights, like stars can be observed, and sometimes bright colored lights. Just allow it all to move into and then out of your frame of observation. Many people, when they first relax into a meditation, see different forms of eyes looking back at them. A bit unnerving the first time I will admit. Just remember that everything you experience is created by you, for your emerging awareness into the expanded human that you are becoming.

Meditation can be as easy as listening to a piece of music that takes you out of your everyday state of thinking and lulls you into a relaxed somewhat hypnotic state. A long walk by yourself in nature can do the same thing. There is no established right form of mediation, just do what feels good to you and your experience will be perfect. I highly recommend trying to make mediation part of your daily routine. Just go easy on yourself if it doesn't happen how you expect it to the first few times. Keep at it, and I guarantee you won't be sorry.

Spending time Alone

Giving oneself the permission to have *me time* is a difficult thing for most westerners to do. It is an important practice however, and should be given very serious attention especially when someone is ill and trying to recover from disease. As you take your body into new energy patterns, there will be shifts that will be felt physically and emotionally. It is key to listen to your body during this time of recovery and treat it well. That means paying attention to energy levels, and not over taxing yourself if you feel tired. For example, you will know when to take a walk because you will feel like doing it—it will appeal to you. If you don't feel like taking a walk, listen to that, and choose another time. Apply this test to pretty much everything you are doing in the run of a day. The recipe is to be present and act on how you feel in the moment.

Do not be around people you do not feel like being around. You know who I mean, the ones who tax your energy field. It's okay to do what feels good to you. This is loving yourself. Putting yourself first. That means staying home when others are pressuring you to go somewhere. That means not answering the phone when you do not want to talk. That means telling people that you are spending a lot of time by yourself so that you can heal and that you appreciate them respecting this. It's all about putting your needs front and center. The courage to do what is best for you.

As you move through all of the physical and emotional changes that will occur as a result of new focus and circumstances, you will feel a lower level of energy at times. A diminished ability to engage with people in the way you used to. This will get better over time, and your energy levels will come back up as you recover, but in the meantime, you need to pay attention to what feels good for you.

I went through various periods where I would just get up and do minimal amounts of everything. If I felt like sitting on the couch and reading, I did. If I did not want to travel to see family members during holiday times, I told them I would not be coming. I really did need the alone time to process all that was happening on so many levels. Stay focused on your body and emotions and be aware of all the situations that can take you out of your healing zone.

Chapter 10.
SOUND THERAPY

It is a simple concept to understand that, when the body is ill, it is out of harmony. It is out of balance. At the cellular level, we are all dancing, vibrating atomic particles. Sound healing is based on the principle of resonant entrainment. That is, when two or more objects are vibrating in the same field and come together—or attune—they begin to vibrate together, shifting to a harmonic resonance, and begin to vibrate identically.

When the body is diseased, it is out of harmony, therefore the vibration is out of tune, so to speak. To heal the body, balanced sounds at intervals are applied to the body and the energy field in order to harmonize and tune any vibrational imbalance that has come about due to illness, injury, or plain old stress. Sound projected into the diseased body can correct the discord and bring the body back into vibrational alignment.

I used sound in various ways to affect my own healing. I often toned, especially to align my chakras, which aligns your energy body. You can find ample ways to be guided with this by going to YouTube. Humming is great also. The use of ohm as a mantra—that is singing it over and over—can be extremely peaceful and brings the body into a state of resonance. The goal is to align your body with the earth, which resonates at its own vibrational level. Since we are all connected to the earth, this brings us all in perfect harmony. Sound is a universal language, and we will all learn to give it more attention and use it in new ways as we move forward.

The majority of these methodologies I used in order to heal myself fall mainly into the category of hands-on or *tangible* practices—ones that I felt I could easily and understandably use to bring my body into a state of physical balance. The more esoteric—yet equally valuable—practices that I would incorporate on an ongoing basis are discussed in the next part of my story. These experiences deal more with the spiritual journey that unfolded in the course of my adventure.

Part 2:

THE JOURNEY

My getting breast cancer actually started many years ago. However, it was only in the last few years that I understood this. It started when I was eight years old, when my mother died suddenly. I can say this is the first clear memory of childhood that I hold. It was very sudden, and quite devastating. This experience created a horrific fear of death in me that lasted until about eight years ago. I only slept for a small part of the night for a good three years after she died.

When I reached my teens and developed physically, almost immediately I had problems with my breasts. They seemed to always be speaking to me in some way, whether I experienced discomfort, or hormonal fluctuations, and ultimately, I began to get cysts, then developed ropy fibrosis. I saw many doctors over many years regarding all these anomalies and had tons of exams, ultrasounds, etc., all trying to ensure there was nothing serious going on. So you see, I was creating the outcome that manifested into cancer all along. This is obvious to me now. The fear I was holding vibrated over a long period of time until it came into the physical energy and showed up as cancer. A culmination so to speak, of a long period of thoughts and emotions around a particular fear. There is much that needs to come forward in this day and age for people to understand the relationship around the emotional body and how it creates the energy which determines physical events. Nothing happens in the physical that is not first created in the energetic fields of thought and emotion. You have heard the phrase *your thoughts create your reality*. Well it's true. They do. I have come to know this up close and personally from my profound experience of creating cancer and then removing cancer from my physical body. I did it by understanding how energy works. I did it by changing my thoughts. I did it by letting go of fear. I did it by allowing my emotions to be expressed. I did it by trusting my body. I did it by putting myself first. I did it by moving into joy. I did it by loving myself. And you can too.

Chapter 11.

11:11

This journey started gaining momentum about eight years ago, and if I could state honestly what was the first recollection I have around things metaphysical or spiritual coming to me in a connected and consistent manner, I would have to say it started with 11:11. I have always had interesting dreams and other worldly experiences from time to time. They were usually noted with interest and then tucked away in the back of my psyche, apparently to be brought forward now as a more complete understanding of life, the universe and everything as it unfolds for me and of course by extension, the entire planet. I am only one of the seven billion people who are waking up on this planet. My story is to help those not yet there to understand and appreciate their respective journey. A journey the whole world is undertaking at this time.

Eight years ago, I started seeing 11:11. *Everywhere!* First it was always on a digital clock. I would see it both morning and evening, and I could never recall having noticed any other time of the day in between. Then I saw it on billboards, on a license plate, on a bus stop, houses, the total amount on a receipt. Anywhere and everywhere it seemed to mock me. I found it interesting at first, then it became such an overwhelming synchronicity that I could not ignore it as an anomaly anymore. Then I started waking up to it every night. I can clearly remember waking up every night for a whole week at 11:11. I was frustrated to the point where I stated out loud:"I am not getting the message, so you had better send me another one!"So for the next whole week I woke up a 1:11. The universe has a great sense of humor.

One of my daughter's finally Googled it, and found out that there is quite a lot of information around 11:11. Millions of people were seeing it at the same time I was. I researched it online, and found there were quite a number of sites dedicated to this phenomena. The overarching explanation for this experience, is that it is a pre-coded cellular wake up call. Everyone is encoded to become more aware at this time in the planet's history, as there is a consciousness revolution going on. That is at the heart of the 2012 timeline being the end of an era. From 2013 on, we are headed into a new era of consciousness that will take us from mind-centered awareness into an era of heart-centered awareness. A golden age. This will be a time where humans evolve tremendously by waking up to the awareness of themselves as an energy with vast universal knowledge within them that comes from the heart/intuition part of them while still inhabiting a body that used to rely solely on the mind/ego. This is a time of the marriage of those two forces in the human body with the heart in full control and the mind subservient to the vaster awareness of the heart. An awareness of the limitlessness of our being and the ever-expanding ability we have to create in the universe.Everyone can feel the change the world is currently undergoing, and it is pretty exciting—at least for those brave enough to consider such ideas, and break the patterning that holds them in bondage to the old world order. It takes courage to think in new ways, to consider new ideas, new experiences. Most people are fearful of stepping outside of the established accepted construct of con-sensus thinking because they are usually made fun of. I know all about this. If you delve into seeking out information that is available worldwide around these concepts you will be amazed that you never came across it before. It has been staring us in the face since the beginning of recorded time. When you desire to know, you will find it comes to you unim-peded. Everything is changing, and it is all perfect.

Chapter 12.
QUANTUM PHYSICS

The next crazy thing that started coming to me—and while now it seems perfectly appropriate, at the time, it just seemed strange—was a bizarre coincidence of everything relating to quantum physics coming into the realm of my observation. I am a voracious reader and have always been. Since my first book at the age of seven I have always loved the power of words—the magic they can bring. I can tell you now, after reflecting back on all the books that have come to me, there is a beautiful cohesion to all of them, and they have given me a greater understanding of who I am here to be. There are no coincidences in the universe, and every book that has found its way to me has been a piece of the unfolding mosaic or puzzle that is me, and my unfolding into who I am here to be.

I am not that good at science. Anyone who knows me well can attest to this. When the topic turns to math, chemistry or physics, my mind shuts down. I am great at biology. My only redeeming area in science. So imagine my confusion when every book or article I would read had something to do with quantum physics. Quantum theory. All things small. At the micro level. I would pick up what I felt was a historical romance, and in it would be something relating to quantum something. And so it carried on, and I began to see the pattern unfolding, and it was at this point, that I truly started to realize that something more than just the random unusual experience was unfolding. I started to pay more attention. And of course, as I focused more on it, the more it increased. This is the essence of the *law of attraction* that everyone has heard so much about. Whatever your predominant vibration is—that is whatever you are giving your thoughts and your emotions to—will attract to you similar experiences and events.

I then became interested enough to start googling certain aspects of the more interesting parts that I could comprehend, and this led me to a major breakthrough. I came across the *multiple universe theory*, and found that most of the leading theoretical physicists subscribed to this theory. That astounded me, and so I read on. This opened the door to a much more expanded view of the universe and matter in general.

Many synchronistic events will come about as you are seeking your path, and this is always a sign from the universe that you are correctly on your soul's path. I had a particularly fun one happen around the quantum theory stage of my journey. One day my husband, out of the blue, brought home a paper for our twin daughters, who were in grade 11 at the time. It was titled "Fractal Geometry and Chaos Theory". A weighty title and subject matter for the dinner table for sure. I remember afterwards that one of my daughters put it in her school bag—at the time even she did not really know why she took it. About a month later, during her math class they were given a list of ten subjects that they could pick from to do a project on. One of the titles on the list was fractal geometry and chaos theory. The humorous part, as she laughingly described to us later, was the look on her teacher's face when she piped up during class as he was handing this out, saying: "Oh, I happen to have a paper here on that very subject!" He was quite impressed that she had such a paper just hanging around in her backpack. Little did she know why she had put that in her bag—she had forgotten about it until that moment. She went on to do her project on that very subject.

During the same time period, my husband and I went to a summer party at the local yacht club. We enjoy living in an area that boasts a lake, river, and ocean, all within minutes from our house. During the course of the evening, I was chatting with a man new to our area, and he turned out to be one of the deans of the physics department at one of our old and established universities. His area of expertise? Quantum physics and chaos theory. By now I was beginning to be less surprised around these charming coincidences. I was starting to see the pattern unfolding.

Chapter 13.

S E T H

My next breakthrough happened as I was following my interest in multiple universe theory. During the course of tracking down all related subjects to this, I came across an excerpt from a book by *Seth*. It was profound to me in a way that started my search for the meaning of life in our universe in earnest. Seth wrote that earth was a school, and that humans were here to learn how to manage their thoughts—for thoughts created reality—and that we were immortal beings that were limitless. This was a heady and provocative bit of literature for me. I needed to find out more. So I joyfully discovered Seth, who was a non-physical entity channeled through a woman named Jane Roberts, who also happened to be an author. Over nearly twenty years, Seth wrote many books about the nature of human reality and the workings of our universe, and I have read all of them. He was my first metaphysical teacher. Jane Roberts also wrote many of her own books. This was also my first introduction to the subject of channeling, which I will expand upon shortly.

So began a period of intense research for everything metaphysical in content. It was not difficult I can assure you. My desire to know everything around this new subject was so strong that it came to me like the floodgates opening. Since most people by this time have heard of the Law of Attraction, you can imagine that my desire was so intense, that the universe sent it to me in spades. I couldn't get enough of it. It was amazing and profound to me that the magnitude of this information was kept out of the mainstream flow of information and out of the educational systems.If one searched specifically for such information it was absolutely everywhere. Many of the major players in history such as Plato, Socrates, Aristotle, Buddha, Christ, Vishnu, Leonardo de Vinci, Lao Tsu, Einstein—just to name a few—all had awareness of how the universe actually worked, but a great effort had somehow been in place throughout history to confuse and keep the average human in the dark around these profound truths. We are not the body. We are immortal; we are pure consciousness inhabiting a physical body. We are all a piece of source energy called *God* by religion and *All That Is* by others. We are all unique individual parts of one large energy, all here acting out a play, characters in our own drama, created by us, and acted out by us, on the stage of third dimensional reality. We live many lives. For me, this was too large, too all-encompassing to be swept under the rug. To my amazement, I have since found out that not everyone is as interested as I am in knowing that there are many more truths to the universe and our part in it. A lot of people are happy to go along with the status quo, having others in positions of authority—within corporations, governments, and religious orders—dictate to them the level of understanding that they should accept within their minds, allowing others to present them with the degree of choices that are available to them. I found that seeking the ultimate truth around who we are here to be is not for everyone. Many are happy in ignorance. Of course, and I say with all sincerity, it is just fine to choose your own level of comfort around such knowledge. The most important law of this universe is that of free will. I spent a lot of time in the early days trying to educate and convince everyone of this new knowledge. I thought I had to save the world from its ignorance. I was saddened and frustrated by the level of apathy I encountered. But as I moved forward and allowed my own awareness to unfold, I realized that we all have our parts to play on this earth, and I had to respect everyone's right to live their part. And so I relaxed around having to beat everyone into awareness and allowed myself to follow a more natural, intuitive approach to when and who I should engage in conversation around metaphysical information.

There is a great documentary that underscores my experience in a far more visual and thought provoking way. It is the story and documentary film from the movie director Tom Shadyac, who directed such films as Ace Ventura, The Nutty Professor, Bruce Almighty, and Liar Liar. He tells a moving tale of how he had it all and then finds out that he had it all wrong. He too faced his own mortality and, in that surrender, he opened up a whole new vista of opportunity for his enlightenment. He travels the world with a film crew, asking famous scientists, philosophers, and religious leaders the same question: *What is wrong with the world?* You can view this heartwarming and mind-blowing documentary by going to iamthedoc.com.

Over the next five years, I allowed the universe to bring me more and more information around higher consciousness and universal truths. I often wondered why I was so driven to acquire all this knowledge and understanding around so many different metaphysical concepts and theories. That was yet to be revealed to me. I could not get over the sheer volume of books and channeled material that was out there—and all of it with predominately the same message. People from different time periods, different parts of the planet, different *planets*, different languages, religions, etc., all with the same message: *We are more than we currently know. We are limitless beings, eternally experiencing ourselves through separation from—and union with—source energy that is called God by most people on this planet."*

I wondered where it was all taking me. I strongly desired to expand into this beautiful awareness. I wanted to speak with energies that were not focused in the here and now. I wanted to see visions of what it was like in dimensions unlike our own. I desired so strongly to grow, expand myself outside of the five physical senses. This I realized, as time went on, was a great summoning on my part. This was the codes of my destiny unlocking within my physical DNA and catapulting me into a new phase of my life here on the changing Planet Earth.

Everything that a person does in this life is planned meticulously by themselves from the discarnate side of life, in the formless, or in the spirit world so to speak. But free will does prevail, so there can be some changes along the way—always in the now moment—that can make the unfolding of a life plan get a little off track. This is the fluid and fun part of existence; the not knowing how it will turn out once the soul is born into the body and enacting the life out in time and space. You really can't get it wrong, as experience in all forms is the desired result. If you stray off the track of your life plan, you will just take a different road that will ultimately get you to the same place. There are levels that you have set for yourself to explore and ascend, and as each one is reached it unlocks codes within your blueprint or DNA that allows new phases of experience to be drawn to you. And this goes on endlessly. We never get it done. So here I was at a point in my life where I was moving into new levels of awareness and experience. I was ready to move into a new phase. Of course, I did not know any of this at that particular time. This is the awareness I hold now, being on the other side of the experience. I was totally unprepared for what was coming my way. I was as surprised as anyone to find myself suddenly stricken with aggressive breast cancer. My metaphysical theoretical musings had come home to roost. I knew for a certainty that this was my moment of truth. My summoning of the energy that would test me as to my new found awareness. I knew that I had *created my own reality*. I was now being asked to walk my talk. And so my life took a new twist, and I entered into the phase of the healing part of my journey.

Chapter 14.
PSYCHIC SURGERY

I had heard of psychic surgery when I was in my late teens. I remember watching a bit about it on television, and it was called *faith healing* at the time. I remember being quite focused on it for a moment, like I was storing it away for some further use. It came to me periodically as the years passed, just the memory and interest around it. I have always been drawn to esoteric spiritual practices.

A month before I received my diagnosis, my husband and I decided to take our first Caribbean cruise. I had recently become aware that there was something going on in my breast, but because of the many episodes I had experienced in the past around the health of my breasts—cysts, fluctuating fluid levels, fibrosis and such—I was not overly concerned at this point. But I knew this time things were feeling a bit different, and so it was in the back of my mind.

In the early days of our cruise, we noticed a young couple who were working with a British Art Auction Company on the ship. When I say noticed, I mean we literally could not get out of their way. It was like the universe was making sure we would meet. Several times a day we found ourselves meeting them around various parts of the ship, and after a while we just started smiling and saying hello. Antonio was from Switzerland, and his girlfriend, Yulian, was from China. Finally one day, Antonio suggests that perhaps we should all go on a day trip together? I was surprised and pleased to have these much younger people want to spend a day with us. We happily agreed, as they were a very pleasant couple. After a great time swimming at a fabulous beach, and sitting chatting in the sand, we decided to find a restaurant and have lunch.

It was during the luncheon that, out of the blue, Antonio started telling us about a trip he and his mother had taken to the Philippines to see this famous psychic surgeon named Jun Labo. His mother had a fallen bladder and needed to have it put back in the correct position in the body. Antonio was amazed at Labo's ability to reach inside a person using only his hands—making an opening much like a regular surgeon would do with a scalpel, only he used just his fingers. How he could remove tissue and tumors and manipulate the interior workings of the body and then close it up with a touch of his hand. Antonio told us that, while he had been prepared ahead of time for what was to happen, he was amazed at the amount of blood that came out during the procedure; he almost fainted as a result. He also told me that his mother enjoyed many months of renewed energy after her visit to Jun Labo.

It was as if I heard a bell ring when he started relating this story. I had instant knowledge that this story was for me, that here was the reason that we had met these people, and that for some reason I was to remember this Jun Labo. I even asked Antonio to spell his name for me and he told me I could find him online.

After this story, it seemed like the floodgates opened on both ends, we started relating some of our spiritual beliefs around life, the universe and everything, and Antonio seemed very interested in all of our metaphysical musings. He said he had thought about such things when he was younger and that he was feeling a hunger to return to such contemplations. The timing was perfect for all of us. We spent a few evenings around the end of the trip talking over dinner about the mysteries of the universe. I am happy to say that we still correspond to this day. Antonio was very influenced with the teachings of "Anastasia" from the series of books called *The Ringing Cedars of Russia*, about the amazing woman living off the grid in Russia, and he is now living in China creating his own artworks, gardening, and planning children with his beautiful partner Yulian. You can view Antonio's art by going to his homepage at www.a–w.ch

It was only after we returned home that I began to realize that I would have get my breast looked at. But for the life of me—no pun intended— I could not bring myself to go have it looked at because I knew that, if the worst were realized, I would not take any treatment. So I decided to have a session with the entity *Veronica*, channeled by April Crawford.

Chapter 15.

CHANNELING

Channeling is the process of communicating with a consciousness that is not in human form by allowing that energy to express itself through a particular individual, who in giving permission for this exchange, becomes the channeler.

The most common form of communication with non-physical consciousness has been with people who have passed on and is more commonly referred to as *mediumship* rather than channeling.

Accessing higher knowledge in order to support spiritual growth and gain greater clarity about one's path through the human experience is usually the reason people seek channeled advice.

I had come across the channel April Crawford serendipitously a couple of years ago. As I stated earlier, I had first been introduced to channeled material a few years before when I encountered Seth, the entity who wrote many books through the author Jane Roberts. I had loved all of the Seth books, dealing mainly with higher consciousness material, and so was quite aware of what the energy coming through April Crawford was all about. *Veronica* is the name April has given to this group energy (more than one consciousness operating in harmony of intention and focus). I listened to everything that was posted on YouTube around them and felt a resonance with their message and a trust that they were very clear in their messages. There is always some distortion with channeled information, and so it is wise to use your own guidance when it comes to what you are hearing—usually a combination of the intellect and intuition will let you know the truth of what you are hearing. April Crawford is a deep trance channel, this is rare, and it means that she vacates the body. That means her consciousness leaves and goes elsewhere, leaving the vehicle free for the energies to come in clearly. April offers private consultations for individuals who would like to speak to the entity Veronica. You can visit her website at www.aprilcrawford.com.

We had taken advantage of this for the first time when my husband had become frustrated with years of acid reflux that he had never been able to cure. He had first engaged traditional medicine in the early years, and had taken pharmaceutical drugs for many years. He eventually realized that he was not dealing with the root of the problem and that he was just compounding his health problems with the drugs. He then turned to naturopathic medicine. This offered a much better solution. He found that his problem was caused by food intolerances and that by ridding his body of these foods, he became totally healed for a while. However, a few years later, he started having new feelings of discomfort that he felt were stomach related again. He decided to talk to Veronica and see if they could shed light on the situation. While they will be quick to tell you that they do not offer medical advice, they will tell you what they see in your energy field. It is your choice as to what action you take from the information they provide you. They see you not as material flesh, but as a vibrating field of energy. They told my husband that his problem was actually not in his stomach, it was in his small intestine and that he had an over abundance of yeast and that this was what was exacerbating the overall problem. And they also pointed out that past lives and your experiences with food in *all your lives* contribute to your experience here in this life. He dealt with the yeast and had total success.

One of my twin daughters had a long standing battle with anorexia. She finally decided to talk with Veronica about this. They told her that she had great difficulty being comfortable in her human body because she does not incarnate often in the physical. She stays in the etheric realms most of the time. As a result she was unhappy with her body and its processes. This resonated on a deep level with my daughter, and she told me it was the first time she had heard something that made total sense to her in terms of how she was feeling. Veronica has had a long ongoing relationship with this daughter and their insight has been instrumental in her having a full recovery.

So now it was my turn to talk with Veronica about myself and what was going on in my body. They would not come out and tell me directly what was wrong with me, but told me it was serious and that I needed a proper diagnosis. So I asked if I could be helped by the psychic surgeon Jun Labo, and they said yes. After speaking with them, I still procrastinated for another month or so before being seen by a doctor. I realized afterwards that I was stalling because, deep down, I knew I would probably not have any treatment if there was something like cancer brewing—and so I was unsure as to what to do. I called Veronica a second time. They were much sterner this time and told me that I needed a diagnosis and that I should not fear having the tests because they were necessary for me to move on.

Ultimately, I went to see the doctor, and because of the advanced state I was in, within four days all tests had been done. The doctors were astounded at the seriousness of my situation and told me that they didn't need to wait for any test results—they said that they would be amazed if it *wasn't* cancer. I now knew, unequivocally, what I was dealing with and so had to make my decisions. There was no room left for further procrastination. My husband and I decided, even before we received confirmation from my biopsy, that we would travel to the Philippines to see the psychic surgeon Jun Labo.

I would like to clarify here that—even though you will read an amazing account of what I experienced in the Philippines with Jun Labo—it is not necessary for a person to have psychic surgery to heal themselves. This was a part of my particular path, and as you will see further on, I did not get a full healing from Jun Labo, for there was underlying emotional work around fear that I needed to let go of. Jun Labo was just step one of my particular journey. I do not want anyone to feel that, because they cannot travel to the Philippines, they will not be able to heal. Nothing is further from the truth. All healing comes ultimately from within. The psychic surgery part of my tale is a great story however, and I include it as a very tangible start of my awareness and guidance around healing modalities beyond what modern science understands.

Chapter 16.
DEALING WITH FAMILY AND FRIENDS

Now came the moment I had to tell family and friends that I had cancer. This was hard. Family and close friends love you and want what is best for you. This goes without saying, and so the diagnosis of a serious illness affects more than just the person receiving the bad news. Family members and close friends are among the things you have to deal with right away in a positive manner to maintain a good level of energy flow so as not to further deplete your energy during a most trying phase of coming to terms with a serious illness.

People, for the most part, mean well when they want to call you, see what is going on, and offer their sage and wise advice. It can be exhausting to talk to so many people during the initial time when you are coming to terms with what is happening to you and your body, and you do not need the extra stress. You have to be candid and to the point without worrying that you are upsetting them by rightfully asking for them to respect your wishes and give you space. Energy is the name of the game, and you do not want to expend what you so greatly need by catering to others who may be projecting their own fears back to you. There are a lot of people who just love to talk about sickness and the drama associated around it. Do not engage with this sort of interaction.

Immediate family members are the hardest, as you are more emotionally tied to them. Understand that all emotion is energy, and the emotions surrounding all the people you interact with and their belief systems are projected towards you and it can have a cumulative effect on your energy if you do not restrict and maintain your own energy field. We have all experienced this in one form or another. Sometimes you can walk into a room where one person is in a bad mood, and everyone can just feel that negative energy; it can affect the whole group dynamic. Or you can get a wonderful feeling when a person who is radiating happiness or joy walks into a room. You just *feel* their exuberance. You have a choice to limit the tone of negativity and encourage an attitude of positiveness from anyone with whom you are interacting with in these early days of adjustment to your new situation.

I was very selective from day one about what I would reveal and talk about with my family. I knew that, at this initial point, they could not understand what was going on within me. I understood that I would receive much resistance to what would appear to them to be the most unorthodox choice for treating the cancer. Aside from certain family members and some cherished friends, most people thought my new beliefs were downright ridiculous. I told my family what I was going to do, asked them to respect my right to do things my way, assured them that I had thought it through and told them that they would just have to trust that I knew what I was doing.

You will face people who will tell you they think you are crazy and ask you to reconsider your decision. You will be told you are not thinking clearly and will be pressured to change your mind and consider traditional medicine. I experienced this. Because of the closeness and trust you share with family members, this can be very emotional and taxing. They are operating from a position of wanting what they think is best for you.

Many people have a fear of death and will give their power over to any external source which they believe knows better than they do about how to heal them. And they will want to convince *you* of this belief. This can be quite intense, and many cave under the pressure. At a time when you are in a state of fear and indecision yourself, it can be tempting to give your own power over to others. Everyone has the right and responsibility to be engaged in their own healing. Now, in my personal situation, it did help that my husband was a tall strong presence who totally supported my decision to undertake my own healing, and fielded quite a lot of the family pressure, which I am eternally grateful for.

It took a little while to get through to people. I was clear with folks that I did not want to hear anything negative and did not want to talk about illness of any sort. I knew that it was important to set a new direction of thought and intention around being healthy, and so any talk of illness was of no use to me. It really did not take that long to get people to do this—everyone for the most part caught on and respected my wishes.In situations like this, those who do not want to comply, do not have your best interests at heart, and you should limit their access to you. Get over worrying about hurting anyone's feelings, you have to put your needs front and centre. This is loving yourself, an important part of the healing process.

It is amazing to me, three years later, that most of the people in my life actually forgot about what was going on with me, and treated me like any other healthy person. They forgot that I had anything wrong with me. I heard this often from people. The success of this is that for the most part, I truly never felt like there was anything wrong with me. And that is how you create a reality of health. You have to *believe* you are healthy.

Fear is the biggest reason behind why people succumb to illness of any sort. Our culture has bred a fear of death into all of us. We have been led to believe that we are a race of beings who are at the mercy of chance, living in a finite world ruled by time. Nothing could be further from the truth. There are dimensions that transcend our time and space continuum. Our consciousness can move into other areas of awareness, outside of the physical body, throughout the universe. Most people are not aware of this as they are stuck in the everyday focus of what they can see from the vantage point of their five senses. And make no mistake, the global elite that currently runs our world has a vested interest in keeping humans enslaved through fear.

While most people are not consciously aware of other dimensions, they actually visit them regularly each night in the dream state. Most people have given up questioning and contemplating the world and how they would like to see it evolve, accepting that things are just the way they are and will never change. Most have given up. They are slaves to desire, comfort, and give their power over to others who they feel better know how to run the world. Governments, institutions, corporations, and militaries have pretty much enslaved the entire planet. All are run by a few people at the top—the global elite—who have been keeping humans distracted from the awareness of their amazing abilities for many millennia.

I *knew* something was coming my way before I actually found out that I had something wrong with me. I did not have an overt knowing or anything like that, more of a subtle thought here and there that told me I was going to have to change something about my life. I could *feel* it coming. I look back and—to be be honest with myself—I can remember having these thoughts. Having no inclination of the drastic experience heading my way, I just ignored these precognitive thoughts as I did not have a frame of reference from which to understand what the thoughts were telling me. So when I received my diagnosis, I knew that the moment of my new journey had arrived. On some level I had been expecting it.

I am a person who has always trusted my intuition. As a child I can remember feeling very strongly that I had to stay strong because I knew something huge was going to happen in my life at some time that would require me to have great courage. I can honestly remember having these strange thoughts around the age of nine years. I would wonder why I had such a strong sense of this, and even remember thinking that I must be going to live through a war or something like that. I had a sense of great destruction around these feelings. So years later, as I have been through my cancer journey, I realize that I was always sensing and align-ing myself for this amazing journey that felt like war in the beginning but ultimately became a peace negotiation.

I have had various curious situations in my life where I have known the answer to things that I did not have knowledge of—whereby the answer or feeling would just come to me out of the blue. I remember one time, when I was about twelve years old, my father and brother were fixing the car out in the driveway. They had the hood up and were troubleshooting what the problem could be. As I walked by them on my way somewhere, I called out...

"It's the *solenoid*."...and then wondered where that came from—I did not have a clue as to what a solenoid even was. And yes, it turned out to be the solenoid switch. They were even more astounded than I was.

I experienced a similar incident when I was in my early twenties and working as a bartender. It was late afternoon and the telephone on the bar rang. As I was heading over to answer it, I somehow *knew* that it was going to be an old boyfriend whom I hadn't seen or heard from in four years. Sure enough, it was him—looking to borrow money I might add! He certainly hadn't changed in those four years.

Another time, again in my early twenties, I had a very vivid dream of two women standing in a room with all glass windows—the only items in this large room being three desks with three telephones on them. One girl was wearing a white dress and the other a red dress. I did not know either one of them. Two years later, I took a job at an international modeling agency. On my first day of work, I was shown into a room with windows on three sides and housing three desks with telephones on them. I was then introduced to the two women with whom I would be working: one of them wearing a white dress, and the other wearing a red dress. I realized in that moment that I could see the future from my dreams. Since then, I have learned to trust my dreams and the messages I send to myself through them.

Therefore, I knew, in a moment of clarity, upon receiving my diagnosis, that I was about to embark on a journey of self discovery unlike anything I had experienced in life thus far. Because, you see, I *knew* that I would not take traditional cancer treatments. I *knew* that I was here to do something different: I was meant to show people that there was another alternative to chemotherapy, radiation, and surgery. I had been preparing for this my entire life. And I *knew* that I would be supported in this by the universe if I could just trust that I would *know* what to do in each and every moment.

I won't say that it wasn't difficult,, especially in the early days. I was very frustrated and a bit scared to deal with all the resistance that I rightly anticipated would be thrown at me from family, friends, and the medical establishment at large. But then again, I have always been an overly ambitious and stubborn personality. But, at that point in my life, I had been given enough awareness around higher consciousness—it had been coming to me for the last five years—that my belief system was very secure in the knowledge that there are energies helping all of us at all times. All you have to do is trust and surrender to their guidance, and it will be yours. I was not disappointed. I gave myself over to the guiding light of universal source and opened myself to hearing and listening to what I should do in each and every moment.

This is called surrender. It is a knowing that whatever is happening in any moment is what is meant to happen and is in your highest interest from a soul evolvement perspective. It is also knowing that, on the higher levels, you are creating your own experience in each and every moment. So I surrendered to whatever was going to be my experience, knowing that I could not avoid it and so embraced and trusted that I was creating this experience for my soul evolvement.

It is my goal to share some specific situations involving this overarching philosophy and give some practical examples. I will try to do this in some sort of chronological order so you can see the progression of how I became more and more confident and secure in my new age approach to healing.

I was given this dire diagnosis—a life threatening illness—and so what am I going to do? At first, I was not sure. I was a bit angry and kind of stressed. I will admit that, but at the same time I was determined to be true to who I was. I have always lived a pretty holistic lifestyle, trusting natural remedies and using exercise, a nutritional diet and herbs to take care of most imbalances in my body. My daughters, as a result of this holistic upbringing, are quite knowledgeable on natural remedies and employ them regularly in their own lives. So this just goes to show that, if it were just a matter of diet (body), I should never have gotten ill in the first place. It goes to show that there are always underlying emotional beliefs (mind) that contribute to a person's overall health.

It is always a matter of balancing body, mind and spirit. So I was not prepared to throw away this belief that I had around being able to balance the body with a natural approach. It would have been a rejection of who I knew myself to be. I was now going to have to walk the talk of my beliefs. I just had to go to a whole new level this time. So I did some talking with my inner self, my soul, and asked for my guides to send me direction on what I should do. And then I listened. This is the most important part—to listen and to trust what you get no matter how esoteric or unusual it may seem to other people. You will get answers when you ask direct questions from your heart to the universe. It will answer. Can you listen?

I am so very fortunate that my husband has been unfolding on this path of enlightenment with me over the past seven years. He has his own way of talking to the universe and has had many interesting and astounding personal experiences of his own that have convinced him that there is a greater awareness beyond what we have been told about life and death.

Being the man he is, he was prepared to allow me to decide my fate and was supportive of whatever I wanted to do. Based on my synchronistic meeting with the man on my cruise and on the information I had already been given twice from Veronica in terms of Jun Labo being able to help me, I decided immediately that psychic surgery would be my first step. Here was leap of faith number one. Travel thousands of miles to a country literally halfway around the world to find a man who can heal with his hands.

The day after I had my biopsy, we left for the Philippines. So, in actual fact, I did not have confirmation of a breast cancer diagnosis until I returned from the Philippines. Ironically it was Jun Labo who first confirmed to me that I had breast cancer. This would be followed up by medical confirmation upon my return.

Chapter 17.

PHYSIC SURGERY IN THE PHILIPPINES/JUN LABO

Once I made the decision to go see Jun Labo, I did some research about him online. You can Google him, there are YouTube videos showing him in action. He is the most famous physic surgeon in the world and has been healing people for almost fifty years. There are books and television shows regaling his abilities. The Germans have published a reader's digest story about him. Burt Lancaster did a show on him in the late seventies. In the producing of this documentary they brought him to a university in the United States, hooked all kinds of wires etc., up to him and then watched him performing his psychic surgery, and filmed it. At the end of the show, Burt Lancaster sums the whole experience up this way:"We don't know how he is doing what he's doing, but he's doing it!"

All who have written about Jun Labo and who have personally seen him in action agree he is actually doing what you see him doing. He is not a fake. There are varying degrees of abilities in physic surgery. Some are not as powerful as others, and of course, as in everything in the world, there are those who are not on the up and up. You have to do your research and use discernment. I felt pretty good about the authenticity of Jun Labo, based on Antonio's story, but still did some research, which proved to be an excellent move, especially as we were traveling to a country that is known for being dangerous, particularly for westerners.

While surfing the net for information on Jun Labo, I happened upon a woman from Oregon who had written a blog about her adventures in the Philippines around physic surgery, in particular about Jun Labo. She has also published a book about psychic surgery in the Philippines. Her name is Jessica Bryan, and you can find all her information on her site at www.psychicsurgery.wordpress.com. Jessica Bryan is an author and book editor who has also guided people on healing trips to the Philippines. I managed to track her down and called her. She was a wonderful person, a great resource, and proved invaluable in our having a problem free visit to this country. Visiting the Philippines is not for the faint of heart. I was guided to Jessica for a reason, and as a result of her experiences, she was able to share with us her wealth of knowledge about safe travel in the Philippines. She recommended that we get in touch with Patrick Hamouy, who in addition to being an expert on macrobiotic eating, is also a guide for people wishing to travel to the Philippines and see Jun Labo. He organized our entire visit. He had us picked up at the airport, booked us into an appropriate hotel for the first night, and arranged for a transport to take us for the six-hour drive to our hotel on the China Sea.

The next morning, he personally accompanied us to the compound where Jun Labo actually lives and conducts his healing. It is heartbreaking to see the abject poverty in the Philippines. There is serious corruption, and it can be dangerous to travel there, especially for westerners. Once we got there and saw how different it was from anything we had so far experienced in our travels, we were extremely grateful to Jessica for her insight and help. She recommended staying in a place by the ocean due to the intense heat. We would need a driver to take us each day to Jun Labo's compound, which was a forty-five minute drive up a huge winding mountain road, the sheer drop from outside our truck window impressed us each day anew. It was a drive that still makes my husband shudder when he thinks about it, but having survived the numerous trips up and down—coming down was no less thrilling—we now take pleasure in showing the pictures to friends, who stare in disbelief at the narrow steep road that goes up into the clouds. It proved to be the best advice, as we had the better part of the whole day after our visits to the compound to sit around and watch the beautiful surf and feeling the somewhat cooling breezes in such a hot stifling climate.

Meeting the Famous Jun Labo

Meeting Jun Labo and seeing his gift for healing was the most life-altering experience my husband and I have had to date. I will try to explain how this man does his work. He has a large room with four facing couches, and people just show up every morning at nine o'clock and sit there and wait for him to come in. You don't have to tell him you are coming, although it is wise to find out if he is at home and not travel-ing, so you don't make a wasted trip. I had done this.

He comes in and sits down and opens a book that resembles the Bible, but was not, I never knew which book it was. He closes his eyes and opens the book at random, and whatever it is he finds there that reso-nates with him, he then writes a passage down on a piece of paper, rips it off, and folds it a few times and puts it in his pocket. An affirmation of some sort is what I took this practice to be. Then he smiles at everyone, and I can tell you he is a most present man when he decides to turn his attention to you. His eyes sparkle and he has a beautiful smile, from his heart, very charismatic with pearly white teeth. He is still a handsome man though he is in his late seventies. He has quite the ego, and thinks very highly of himself. He is also known to be quite kind and is full of desire to help the less fortunate. He has an orphanage that he funds himself. He has run for mayor of his town of Baguio no less than three times, in the hopes of being elected so that he can pass a law limiting the amount of car emissions so that he can help eliminate the horrendous smog that envelopes most of the cities in the Philippines. He is humble in his gift of healing, however; and he is very compassionate.

He continues by motioning all assembled to move over to the benches that are in front of life-size statues of Mary and Jesus. There is an altar, and it all feels like being in a church. Jun Labo states that his healing gift comes from Christ, that he is channeling the energy of the Christ Consciousness—when people of Arab descent come, he channels healing from Rama. He is quite sincere in his statement that all healing comes from Christ and Rama, not from him. He is just the instrument. He takes his responsibility very seriously. He then lights some incense and goes into a lengthy prayer to Jesus about helping him to be able to help his brothers and sisters, and giving gratitude for all that he has been given.

Once this ritual is complete, he ushers everyone downstairs to the room he uses for performing physic surgery. I can tell you that it is not what would be considered a western traditional hygienic operation. What is fascinating is how he works on one person, and then another with no form of disinfectant of any kind—a horrifying thought in any modern hospital—and there is never any complications from having him work on you, such is the purity of the higher vibrations coming through this mortal man.

All of a sudden he goes into trance, and it is very easy to see the difference in his person during this transition. He gets a certain look on his face, his eyes seem very different and he speaks very little and abruptly. Everyone takes off all their clothes except for their underwear, and stand in a lineup. All assembled are only four feet away from the table and so one can clearly see all that transpires. I can only say at this point that there is no doubt whatsoever as to the authenticity of what happens at this moment.

The first person is gestured to lie on the table, and he holds a white sheet up to their body and, somehow, looking through this sheet, shows him what he needs to know, where the illness in the body is located. He then quickly moves his fingers like he is jiggling the skin back and forth and it opens. Blood comes out and also various items such as tumors, blood clots, pieces of stringy skin, like earthworms, and other such biological anomalies.

It has been postulated that a form of magnetic attraction takes place, whereby all diseased and undesired organic material comes to his hands from all parts of the body. He often throws whatever he gets right on your chest or abdomen while he is looking for other stuff. His hands never leave your body. When he has what he is looking for, he quickly touches the area and the skin is all back together like he was never there—except for the blood. There is lots of blood with physic surgery.

When it was my turn, I was of course quite nervous. As I lay down on the table he immediately started moving his fingers around my left breast. I could feel the hot spurt of blood, and I could smell the tangy acrid scent of copper, along with a sickly sweet smell I realized later was the smell of disease. He took out a couple of tumors that day, small ones, and also long pieces of tissue from my abdomen and pelvic area.

I have to say there is no sensation of pain at all; it is more like being tickled. When he is done, he motions you to quickly get up off the table, a nice man with wet towels wipes the blood off you, and you get out of the way for the next person in line to jump up on the table.

All in all it was the most amazing and miraculous—albeit somewhat barbaric—experience of my entire life. It defied all the laws of modern science, yet there it was. I could not deny what I had witnessed and felt along with the others in the room. Where to go from here? My world had been redefined.

My husband had no less an amazing experience, he had decided that he would see if Jun would find anything wrong with him, he had travelled all this way after all, and our guide said it would be a shame to waste the opportunity. So he too had many interesting things taken out of him that day, some cysts, and some blood clots in his legs.

After all are seen and operated on, you meet back upstairs again on the couches, and Jun comes and sits down and tells you what is wrong with you. At no time do you tell him anything about what you are there for. So he was the first person to confirm to me that I had breast cancer. He told me it was traveling, and drew a picture of where it was spreading in the body. He told me he would only know by the end of the treatments whether or not he had gotten all of it. He then told my husband there were a couple of things wrong with his back and groin area that would give him much trouble in the years to come, and that he could take these from him. So we both settled in for the ten day treatments that were required for our particular health issues. Some people only require one treatment; it is different for each person depending on their health situation and life path.

Over the course of the next ten days, I had various organic diseased tissues taken out of my body, one day he removed a very large tumor, and since I usually closed my eyes for the procedure—I found this easier personally, but was enthralled to watch him work on others—he barked at me to *look*, he wanted me to see what he had removed.

At the end of the ten treatments, I knew that he had not totally taken it all from me. He had cleaned me up quite a lot, but it was a few months before I came to realize that my journey involved not just the tangible physical fact of illness in the body, but that the illness is always caused by an underlying emotional belief that is causing the illness, and that to remove the part that was attached in my heart area would have killed me.

Such is the universal knowledge that the entities working through Jun Labo hold, they can see your life path and know when you are ready for healing and when you need to continue your journey on your soul's path to enlightenment. It was not my time for a full healing, but he had helped me tremendously in pulling the cancer back to a place where I had the time to breathe, take stock, and decide what my next move would be.

I was still trusting in the universe to guide me, and my trip to the psychic surgeon was the start of my healing. I know now that psychic surgery is not necessary for everyone to heal, it was just an experience that was perhaps necessary for me personally to experience so that I would have more trust in the non-physical aspect of healing. It certainly helped me have an easier time of it, and I have great respect and gratitude to Jun Labo for his gift and sacrifice in helping so many thousands of people over the years. I will always remember my fantastic trip to the Philippines.

Taking Stock after Psychic Surgery

When I got back from the Philippines, I had to deal with a lot of questions from family and friends about my decision to travel and have psychic surgery. There was much arching of eyebrows, and many people were somewhat skeptical about the fantastic story my husband and I brought home—even though they were kind enough not to say so in words, we could tell they were thinking it! It helps that my husband is a very well-respected engineer, and so people found it harder to dismiss his confirming that this had actually happened. I do think that had I been there by myself to experience the physic surgery, that it would have been dismissed much quicker in people's minds—sad but true. I observed that most people seemed to find it hard to refute my husband's rendition of our experience; they seemed to be more accepting of his words, while I would get the furrowed brow expressions whenever I was relating it. Such is the religion of science in this day and age, that the masculine scientific mind is more accepted as the definitive answer. The need for the power of the intuitive feminine energy to move into its rightful place to bring balance is clear.

I also had to respond to the medical personalities who now had my test results back, and confirmation of my cancer. They were ready to take action, by recommending immediate chemotherapy and radiation, in the hopes of ultimately being able to do surgery. They were totally unaware of the fact that I had different plans.

At this point, I was still unsure of how I was going to proceed. I knew that I would not have chemotherapy or radiation. These were not on the table for me, as I knew I was going to walk the path of healing myself without destroying my body in the process. I had however, not ruled out surgery at this time.

I felt that I should explore the options left open to me, so I proceeded to set up an appointment for a visit with the surgeon. I ended up seeing a female doctor whom I had seen many years ago for cysts in the breasts. Initially I had been scheduled to see another doctor, and for some reason that appointment was cancelled and, like a lot of similar moments, this one turned out to be a perfect fit. I could not have asked for a better outcome.

I remember being somewhat intimidated by her from our first meeting years ago. She had a strong personality and would not see anyone unless they first took her seminar on how to care for the breasts through self-screening. I felt there was synchronicity around her sudden insert as my doctor. I was a bit afraid of our upcoming encounter, as I knew I was going to tell her about my having gone to the Philippines for physic surgery and was anticipating resistance or ridicule around this, if not outright apathy. Imagine my surprise when I told her where I had gone and what I had done, and she replied:

"I know exactly what you are talking about, I have a friend who does psychic surgery in South America. Tell me what he said and what he took." What were the odds? It could not have been sweeter. So after I explained what he did, she said that the prudent thing would be to do some testing and see where we were at. I told her I was not sure what testing I would consent to do, but asked her if she would at some point be available to do surgery should I desire it, and she told me that she would be happy to do whatever I wanted to have done.

Now I had the dilemma of whether or not I should have testing done to see where things were at. It seemed counterintuitive to me, after spending all this effort to clean up my body, to consent to tests that were going to put dyes and radioactive isotopes into my system—not a good thing at all from my perspective.

With much deliberation, I decided it was time to talk with Veronica again. They had a look at my energy and said that Jun Labo had cleaned me up quite a lot, but that it was important that I know exactly where my body was at, and so it was their feeling that I would benefit on some level from having the testing—that it was important to me in moving forward on my path. I was not really happy to hear this and pointed out to them that I felt the testing would be harmful. They told me to go into the tests with a positive intention for all to come out well, not to have any fear around it. This is exactly what I did. They put dyes through me to see if there was anything in the organs, liver, etc.. They also did a bone scan. For both of these tests, I meditated while they were going on, and actually felt quite euphoric especially during the half hour bone scan; I could actually feel the support and help I was receiving from energies around me. As a result of my keeping my spirits positive around the testing, they came back totally clean, they could find nothing—which I think surprised them all. Being surprised was something they would have to get used to! I did end up having a full body rash and was quite itchy for three days from all the chemicals they put into my body. In hindsight, I now understand the importance of going through the biopsy and all the subsequent testing, as this documented, scientifically, exactly what type of cancer I had along with the severity of it in order that I would have solid data when it came time to write my book. I made up my mind that those tests were the last ones I would have. I also decided that there would be no surgery.

Chapter 18.
SYNCHRONICITY

The role of coincidence, also known as synchronicity, plays a very important role in the understanding of guidance and the unfolding of one's awareness of the spiritual or metaphysical path.

Synchronicity is when you see something one day, and then see it again in a different place soon after, or hear about it from a person in some conversation, etc. Any repetitive occurrence that shows up in a relatively short time frame is a sign of synchronicity. So meeting a person you have never met before one day, and then hearing a friend mention that very same person the next day can be an example of this. Hearing someone speak of a book, and then seeing it on a bookstore shelf soon after, or having it show up on an internet site is another example. It can also show up as numbers, such as 11:11, like I experienced, or as 444, 555, etc. My sister in law had quite a run of sevens in her life. She would continually see 777 or 7777. She was quite enjoying this run of lucky 7s as she termed it. You can also Google the meaning of numbers, as they hold clues to what you are trying to show yourself by bringing that particular synchronicity to your conscious awareness.

These synchronistic experiences are the universe talking to you. They are showing you that you are on track and paying attention. This is you being aware of the connectedness of patterns unfolding in your experience. It is fun and affirming. I love it when I experience synchron-icity, I feel like I am getting a pat on the back from the higher part of myself.

Chapter 19.
R E I K I

After I received the clean bill of health regarding the rest of my body, I set about with great determination to heal myself with whatever healing modalities presented themselves to me. I was now feeling the effects of all that had happened to date, and so my energy was quite low compared to my normal levels. I intuitively felt that it was a time to take it easy, not push myself. Along this journey I would reach a state where one thing would be completed and then something new would always show up, in the form of a person, email, book, event, dream or inspiration. Such was the level of synchronicity that I was experiencing. The universe talked to me daily in some form or the other. On a random visit to my local garage, I met a woman who started talking to me out of the blue about higher consciousness and invited me to an event she was organizing with this spiritual friend of hers. I accepted, knowing that it would be interesting if nothing else. It was here that I met my next guide, Elizabeth, who is a reiki master. Reiki is a form of energy healing by which a person moves universal healing energy through another's body by use of their hands in order to facilitate a positive change in that person's energy field. The intention set by both the practitioner and client can help the level of healing received. So I started seeing Elizabeth twice a week.

I could really feel the difference in my energy after having a session with her. At this time, I felt like I was very fragile and etheric in some way, like I was drifting or floating through my life. After having the reiki done on me, I felt more alive. We also spent time talking about what the emotional under-pinnings of my illness could be.

While she was operating during the healing sessions, Elizabeth would often receive messages from her non-linear self, and one day she told me she heard a clear voice telling her that I needed a *core pattern reading* from a person she knew in Toronto—a woman who called herself Anandashakti. This was to send me on a totally different direction with my healing path. While I continued on with Elizabeth and the reiki sessions for a few months longer, I was set to open up a brand new experience which was to be nothing less than fantastic. My time with Elizabeth was beautiful, healing and restful. You can connect with her by email at maptoevolve@gmail.com, or directly by phone at 1-902-221-3830.

Chapter 20.
ANANDASHAKTI

Anandashakti is a woman who teaches a series of healing modalities which includes her own style of yoga and various other Indian Vedic practices. You can view her online at www.sananda.ca. I contacted her for a core pattern reading as suggested by Elizabeth.

This is a specific reading that is achieved when a medium allows themselves to be used as a conduit for an energy to come through and pinpoint the specific life pattern that is repeating itself and wanting to be resolved. There are many well recognized angels residing in the spiritual realms, such as Archangels Michael, Gabriel, and Raphael. One of the lesser known but just as powerful is Archangel Metatron. This is the energy that Anandashakti channels when she is performing these core pattern readings. This was another synchronicity for me, as years ago when I first started meditating, the very first time, I had a vision behind my eyes of an electric blue ibis-headed Egyptian, which is the symbol of the Egyptian God Thoth, who at the higher levels is Metatron. So I booked an appointment with her. This proved to be a most interesting experience. It is done over the telephone. First I will tell you of this most unusual experience with Ananda, and then I will tell you the even more amazing reason why I met this woman. Much was meant to unfold between her and I.

Over the telephone, she asked me to take a few deep breaths and relax while she moved into the spaciousness reserved for her to bring this forward. She did some beautiful toning and breathing, and after a time she said she was ready to bring forward the information. She spoke for almost an hour, first describing what was going on in my body, where the disconnect was coming from, explaining that my body could not hold the energy; it was like a house with an open window— no matter how often I heated the house up, the energy would leak out through the window. She told me that that I had an underlying mood of despair and unworthiness that was very deep. Then she was shown the particular life that was responsible for my current problem in this life.

She described a life where I was sexually abused by a father and three brothers, from the age of five years old. She related how I had no safe place to call my own because the mother was consciously choosing not to see the abuse. Because I felt I was not safe in my body, at the age of fourteen, I killed myself by refusing to eat or drink. A very heavy life that was described in detail.

After this part of the reading, she commented on the meaning of why I chose this life. While this was, on the surface, a very dramatic and sad life, there was also much for my soul to gain from this experience. Furthermore, I would know, at a future point, why I had chosen to be on the receiving end of this. It was explained that, while I had an awareness of this sadness in my soul, that I needed to go to a deeper level at this time.

It was a poignant and revealing experience, and while there is always some distortion around such information, I felt that I had gone to the heart of the matter and that, in and of itself, gave me confidence that I had received a very important piece of the puzzle as to why I was on this journey. This experience led me to understand that cells retain all memory from all lives, and that a person can have trauma from other lives still encoded in their cells, so not all problems manifesting in the physical are coming from the current life. Around this time, I was introduced to the work of Caroline Myss, the well-known medical intuitive and author.

Caroline Myss is a woman who has a gift that shows her what illness is going on in a person's body and where it is coming from. She sees the energy of this from a multidimensional perspective at the quantum level. Her understanding of illness and how it can come from other lives was quite an eye-opener for me. According to her, we squander much of our energy by leaving it in past events and wounds we have experienced in current and past lives. We have not let go of them yet, and so our energy is still keeping it in vibration. It is important to let go of talking about past hurts and painful experiences and forgive all the people involved and to call our energy and spirit back to us in the present moment. The NOW. This integrates the release on all levels, not just this life, but the concurrent lives that are being lived in other places and times.

Facing the fears we harbor for disease and illness—and trusting that all will be well if we just discontinue to hold these thoughts and feelings in vibration—is key to healing yourself. Learn to love yourself, unconditionally. Just let go. Let go of self-judgment. Let go of having to be in control. Love yourself for your imperfections, and realize all experiences in all lives are for the purpose of feeling contrast. To know the full experience of joy, one must experience deep sadness. Everything you have ever lived has been designed by you for the purpose of experiencing life as a contrast. In all its diverse moments. Nothing is right or wrong. It is only your perception of an experience that makes it a good one or a bad one. Surrender the need to pass judgment on anything. Only then can your energy effect a full healing. The alternative healing modalities, like diet and supplements, are a help but not enough on their own. Again, it is a combination of body, mind and spirit. Let go of fear. This is well documented with people who engage in past life regression and are instantly healed upon remembering the past life situation that is responsible for their current life problem or illness.

I did try having a past life regression done on a couple of occasions in order to move into the life that is causing the current illness and release the trauma from it, but to no avail. I was not successful in going into a hypnotic state, meaning that this was not my path. Acceptance of what works and what does not is key, as everyone's path takes a different road. I will get back to my adventures with Ananda, but first I must set the stage with an explanation regarding another famous healer.

Chapter 21.
HEARING ABOUT
JOHN OF GOD

TAMANA

During my trip to the Philippines I had met a woman from France who was also there to see Jun Labo, and it turned out that she had a rare form of bone cancer, and was shrinking in size, yet no doctor had been able to diagnose her. We struck up a friendship of sorts, and still communicate to this day. She was the first person to mention John of God to me. I had a vague memory of having heard about such a person at some point in my past, but it certainly was not in my conscious mind at this point, that is, not until Tamana mentioned him to me. She told me she had done research on two famous healers and been torn as to whether she should go to Brazil to see John of God, or to the Philippines to see Jun Labo. Jun Labo won out. It proved to be the right choice in my opinion, as Tamana later made the journey to visit John of God (twice) and is now fully healed as a result of her following her heart and intuition. She is currently a FARA therapist and you can view this healing modality at www.faradarmani-france.com. My meeting with Tamana and hearing about John of God proved to be part of my continuing path.

It is important to understand that it is not necessary for a person to go to John of God to be able to heal themselves. Much like psychic surgery, this was a part of my particular journey and is not a necessary requirement for a person to heal. I would like to add, however, that you can find official guides online who are sanctioned by John of God. They will ask you to send your picture over the internet and they will take your picture in front of John of God, and the entities will determine what they can do for you, and you can have a certain amount of healing done from a distance. You can research this online. I saw many people doing this while I was there, and there is much help to be had this way, as the entities transcend time and space and can work on you from any-where. John of God is the vessel they speak through to communicate with us.

For those of you who have not heard of John of God, let me fill you in on this amazing man. No less fantastic than Jun Labo, yet in a totally different way does he help heal millions. This man is also gifted with the ability to have energies heal through him, and while this is primarily what he did in his younger years—helping people to heal—he was guided to take this to a whole new level as time went on. You can Google him for more information, the most reliable site is www.friendsofthecasa.com.

John of God has built a spiritual hospital in the small community of Abadiana, Brazil, at the behest of the spiritual entities that incorporate through him. They advised him in the 1970s to build this compound in a small town on a mountain founded on a bed made of quartz crystal, which helps facilitate the ease of entities communicating with the lower vibrational density of the earth plane. These entities that come through John of God pretty much run this entire operation by way of the com-plete surrender that John of God allows in their use of his physical vehicle in order to communicate all their wisdom and healing energies to all who ask it of them.

There are many volunteers, people of high spiritual awareness that transcend any specific religion, who are happy to facilitate the dictates of the entities that come through John of God. While he does perform some psychic surgery, the majority of the healing that is done in Abadiana is very much different that that of Jun Labo. I will elaborate more on my trips to Brazil, but for the moment I want to give you an understanding of my interesting synchronicity around John of God and Ananda. It is important for all to see how well-guided I was during this journey, and it is my hope that most of you will agree that the amount of what people call coincidence was way beyond what most would consider normal. There is no such thing as coincidence in the universe, and I know this now with all my heart.

I was scheduled to have my core pattern reading with Ananda on a Wednesday. On the weekend just before this, I had been giving some thought as to whether or not I should go to Brazil and see John of God. This had not really been on my mind; it seemed to suddenly come up in my attention. I chatted with my husband about it, and he said that he had felt all along that we would probably go there since hearing about him from Tamana. He felt this more strongly than I did at this point. Personally I was not getting a solid feeling around it, and so decided that I would just put the thought out to the universe and see what came of it. I was beginning to learn this skill. To clearly ask for something and then see what comes your way. With this thought in mind, on the Sunday night prior to my session with Anandashakti, I asked the universe whether I should go see John of God?

The very next day I received an email from Tamana, (had not heard from her in a couple of months) telling me she was off to Brazil to see this John of God! That was indication number one. Then in speaking of it with Elizabeth while having reiki on Tuesday, she said: "Let's ask the tarot." Tarot cards are a form of divination, and have been used throughout time. She pulled out a deck of tarot cards and asked me to set my question to them. So again I asked whether I should go to John of God. The two cards I pulled were *Seer* and *Crystals*. Elizabeth laughed. "That seems pretty clear to me!" That was indication number two. But the most clear and amazing indication came from a seemingly random event. The tapestry of connecting threads that binds all of our daily lives and multiple existences has a beautiful order at levels far beyond our conscious understanding of what we term chance and is in reality destiny. There is a recent television series that clearly and artistically depicts this core connection of all people and events. It is called "Touch".

The day before I was to have my core pattern reading with Ananda, I received my first email from her—she had put me on her email list. Now you have to understand, I have no prior knowledge of this woman other than speaking with her for a few minutes to schedule a time for the core pattern reading. Imagine my amazement when I receive an email describing her life changing trip to Abadiana, Brazil and her acceptance as a qualified guide to bring people to see John of God. She advertised her upcoming scheduled trip to take interested persons in November of the year. I took this as a clear sign that I should go and see John of God. After asking the universe what I should do, I had received three solid indications around it, within three days. The only fly in the ointment for me was that it was middle June, and I did not think I should wait until November to go to Brazil. I felt I should go as soon as I could.

On Wednesday, after I had finished my core pattern reading with Ananda, I told her about my desire to visit John of God, and how excited I was that she was a guide but that I did not think I could wait until November.

After hearing me out, she exclaimed with barely contained excitement. "This is so strange," she said, "that you should call me with this, as I originally had a trip planned for early August, but we were two people short." She told me she would call me back in a short while, and sure enough, two hours later she called me to say that if my husband and I were willing we would all go in August. She too realized that there was energy around us going to Brazil together at this specific time. Such are the ways that seemingly unrelated circumstances line up to produce patterns, if we are willing to pay attention to the signs. We are always divinely guided; we just don't often trust it enough to place our faith in the unfolding of it. There were too many coincidences around this whole experience for me not to see that I was being well-guided, and so I surrendered to the next phase of my journey.

Brazil and Meeting John of God

Getting to Brazil was somewhat easier than going to the Philippines, but still presented some challenges. Not as easy as taking your passport and flying to Europe or the United States. They required a visa, and we needed to send our passports to Montreal to acquire one, so the timing was a bit tight, but it all worked out on time, and we received a ninety-day visitor's visa.

We flew to Atlanta, Georgia, the first day and then caught a direct overnight flight to Brasilia. Brasilia is an interesting city that was originally designed and built in the shape of a bird—one of the few cities in the world to be constructed from scratch. It took four years to build and has a population of four million people. A driver from our *Pousada* (the Brazilian word for our accommodations) met us at the airport, and after an hour and a half drive through the countryside, we arrived in the small town of Abadiana.

We were warmly met by our hosts, Catherine and Russell, owners of the Pousada Luz Divina. Ananda and the other two members of our group were to arrive later that day, but due to unforeseen difficulties, they ended up being caught in airports for an additional two days. Our hosts took the time to show us around the compound, which was only a few blocks away. My husband and I arrived on a Sunday afternoon, and by Tuesday night Ananda had finally arrived—a bit harried but accepting of whatever reasons kept her from being there at the same time as us. This was the first time we had met in person, and I was immediately taken with her warm and caring nature and her profound spiritual commitment. She was efficient in taking stock of what we wanted to ask the entities, and after a lovely supper and a visit in the gardens outside, we all went to bed. The next morning, we were up and ready on time to head off to our first meeting with John of God.

The workings of the spiritual hospital known as Casa Dom Ignacio De Loyola are steady and smooth, thanks to the vision of the entities and the organization of the volunteers who oversee and carry out their wishes and dictates.

Dom Ignacio De Loyola is the principal entity that incorporates through John of God, and he is about four hundred years old by linear earth time. The entities coming through John of God do so in the same manner as I earlier described with the entity Veronica channeled through April Crawford. However, there are a host of additional entities that come through John of God each and every day, and sometimes no one is sure who is in the body at a given time. There are regulars who show up, and they are mostly known to the translators/volunteers. Most of the entities have been doctors or healers of some sort in their previous incarnations. There are pictures and paintings of various entities from their earthly lives displayed along the walls of the Casa.

Regularly throughout the year—every Wednesday, Thursday and Friday—John of God shows up early in the morning to allow himself to be of service to the thousands of people who show up each week to present themselves in front of him to receive guidance and/or spiritual healing from the entities. There is a morning session, a lunch break, and then an afternoon session.

People fly in from all over the world, stay in one of the numerous pousadas built around this spiritual hospital, or arrive on one of the many large buses that come from all over Brazil and other parts of South America. People are asked to wear white when going in front of the entities as this allows them to see your energy body more clearly.

There are translators available to write your question out for you, for John of God only speaks and understands Portuguese and so all questions and answers are in this language. Everyone lines up, there is quite a system to this depending on whether you are there for the first time, second time, etc., and while it did seem confusing the first day, we quickly caught onto the system and saw it was quite ingenious in its unfolding. Nothing about this operation could be considered normal by our linear and western sensibilities, so it is best to just keep an open mind and reserve all criticisms, a good attitude is beneficial to your overall experience and healing.

Spiritual Operation

My first time in front of the entities was quick, and this is the usual experience for most people. The entities literally start working on you the moment you decide you are going to Brazil. They work from a place outside of time and space and so are not bound to our idea of time. I could feel them working on me before I left Nova Scotia—I noticed a shift, a new feeling that I had not felt before, a subtle knowing that they were there. They know well ahead of you appearing before them in the

line what they have in mind for you. They listen to the question, but for
the most part the answer is already there, and they quickly move onto the
next person, as there are many to see in the three hour sessions. So I was
told immediately:"Operation this afternoon. Next!"They said the same
thing to my husband.

A spiritual operation is different than psychic surgery. John of God
does perform actual surgeries in front of the whole congregation waiting
in line; I have seen this up close and personal on two occasions. He uses
a scalpel to do them—with no anesthetic I might add—and his patients
experience zero pain. Much like psychic surgery, he will open the person's body and remove whatever needs to be removed; there is blood,
and then he will sew them up. They are then taken to a recovery room
nearby, and most heal much faster than average. A couple of days and
usually there is no sign that he was even there.

The majority of healing's are done via a spiritual operation. This is
done in a specific room. Everyone who has been told to show up, sit
side by side along rows of pews. There are volunteers who manage these
rooms by asking everyone to close their eyes. They then proceed to voice
prayers in a soft lulling monotone, mostly in Portuguese, but sometimes
in English while the entities work on the entire group from the etheric
realms. Energy work and healing is done from the higher levels of vibration and is then moved into the density of matter. You can literally *feel*
the energy moving through the room. Now I am a person who does not
feel energy as easily as others do. My husband feels energy much more
immediately than I do. He can hold a crystal and feel it buzz and tingle
in his hand. I can sometimes feel this, but not always. He can instantly
feel such subtle workings especially when he meditates.

I was a bit anxious and overly attentive during my first spiritual
operation—not to mention extremely warm, for a regular day in Brazil
is a scorcher for any Canadian—and while they have plenty of fans, they
do not have air conditioning at the Casa. I was very much aware of the
feeling in the room, a heightened electrical energy was pervading the
whole room. At one point, I felt something push me suddenly right in
the area of my solar plexus. There was no one touching me on either
side, and so it startled me. I will never say that I have experienced or felt

energy unless it is so. I am always truthful with myself. I could feel subtle internal workings that seemed a bit foreign to my body, but that was really the extent of my experience during the actual thirty-five-minute operation. When it was finished, they asked everyone to go outside to certain designated areas that were oriented to your spoken language and they gave us very specific instructions as to how we were to spend our next twenty-four hours.

The volunteers are very intent about having you understand the enormity of what has just happened to you. Some people have the equivalent of four or five surgeries during this thirty-five-minute ordeal. The entities can perform beyond the constraints of third dimensional abilities, and so a person's body has undergone quite a transformation and healing during this operation. They are adamant that no one walks back to their pousada, even if it is only a couple of blocks. They stress that no one would get up off a traditional hospital bed after undergoing a regular surgery and walk home, and so they stress that one must accept the seriousness of doing such a thing even though they cannot physically see the surgery. I could relate to this perhaps more than the average visitor due to my experience in the Philippines. The first night after Jun Labo had taken tumors out of me, my body had quite a reaction. I felt quite off, was shaking like I had the chills, almost had what I perceived to be a panic attack—I was a mess. My husband said he felt my symptoms were like the body being in shock. My guide told me the next day that the body and mind have no logical explanation for what it was seeing and feeling and so reacts quite violently to the experience. After a couple of days, my body became used to the sessions, and I felt just fine.

In Brazil, I took their advice very seriously and followed their instructions to the letter. A person is required to go directly to bed wearing white for twenty-four hours. You are not even allowed to get up to eat—someone must bring you your meals. I can see why this is so important. Not only is your body dealing with the change in energy and matter, but also they continue to work on you during this twenty-four hour period. You are almost in a trance-like state. The time seems to pass quickly, like you are in a lucid dream state. After the twenty-four hour period is reached, you go in front of the entities again, and they either schedule you for another operation or they tell you that what they have done for you is complete for now.

My second trip in front the entities was a bit of a shocker. It is important to understand that from my first time in front of them—which took all two seconds—to my second time, there had to have been close to 2,500 people go before them.

I had an inspiration around an endeavor that I wanted their feedback on, and so I asked a question relating to this. They seemed to ponder it and asked who would facilitate this undertaking I had asked about. When I replied that I would be the one undertaking this, they kind of yelled at me. While I am sure there was no actual yelling, that is how it felt. They abruptly told me that I could do nothing until I had dealt with what was going on in my breast, and that I needed to get my head around it and be practical. There was a tough love, impatient feel to the tone of how it was said, and then I was abruptly dismissed. My husband came after me, and they told him—in a much kinder tone—that it would be good if we could stay for another week.

Feeling like a chastened child, I went outside and immediately burst into tears. Ananda was with us the entire time in front of the entities, so she heard the whole thing. She was very empathetic, but I am not one to show much emotion in front of others—something I am still learning to let go of—and so ended up railing at the powers that be in some little chapel nearby, and crying my eyes out.

I realized later—and have come to realize this on many occasions since—that such situations are a great release of energy and can open up new pathways for new and more productive experiences. I am sure this was their intention in giving me ruthless compassion.

I would like to underscore for those who have not yet picked up on this: How does John of God keep straight what ailment is in front of him? I was only in front of them once before, and the second time I did not mention anything to them about my breast. For them to so clearly articulate what my problem was after only seeing me the once, about 2,500 people ago is nothing short of miraculous. Such is the way of the etheric realms and their abilities to see beyond what we can see in the physical.

I was in front of the entities twice more, and they prescribed crystal beds, and a trip to the waterfall but no more operations. I will get to crystals beds and the waterfall in a moment. My last visit in front of the entities, on a Friday afternoon, was much more loving and humorous.

I asked them where I was at, and they replied what they had done for me was complete for now. They smiled and told me to go into the other room for a blessing. As I turned to leave, I heard them say, "You'll be back." Surprised, I turned back and asked, "When?" They smiled. "You'll know." This was curious to me, because I did not have any plans to return, this trip was expensive enough! But the most curious thing unfolded; on our return trip, my husband and I had a layover in Atlanta between flights, and so, out of boredom, I happened to look at my Brazilian visa. I had purchased two ninety-day visas. Only I noticed that mine was now valid for two years. My husband looked at his, and it said ninety days. He was quite astounded by this, as he told me that he remembered looking at both of them when they first arrived, and that they were both ninety-day visas. I was to return to Brazil later that year, but at this particular time I had no such plans.

Crystal Beds

One of the most magical and therapeutic healing tools that the Casa offers are their crystal beds. These were designed and built from the instructions given through John of God from the entities.

There are seven beautifully faceted crystals matching the colors of the chakras inside the body. Chakras are the energy portals within a person's energetic body. I have a section, further on, that explains in more detail the miraculous abilities of crystals. These crystals have a laser type light shone through them as they are positioned to line up with your chakras as you lay on the bed. A cloth is laid over your eyes, and beautiful music is played while you mediate under these amazing crystals.

There are many remarkable stories surrounding the experiences that happen in these crystal beds. I can share with you my husband's first experience as he had quite a dramatic one. My husband has been beside me as I've walked my healing road, a very supportive partner, who has enjoyed the various experiences right along side of me. So he really had no expectations when going for his first crystal bed. I might add that I have never seen my husband cry in the many years we have been together, he is a very quiet and logical man with an air of integrity about him. When he described his crystal bed experience I was pretty astounded.

He described it all as starting out nicely, quiet and relaxing with beautiful music playing. His mind started pleasantly drifting and then—all of a sudden—he recalled this childhood situation involving a white kitten that he had found and brought home. Excited and full of love for this little creature, he showed it to his parents, but it was full of worms and died. As a result of the trauma associated with this he had buried that unpleasant experience, not to recall it until this moment. He said he was bawling like a baby, and then all of a sudden it felt like he was rocking from side to side. He fell into a pleasant lull with this motion, and then it stopped. He remembered thinking that was so soothing that he didn't want it to stop. Then he started rocking in the opposite direction, back and forth. He had quite the release from his emotional body during this first session.

A typical crystal bed session lasts for twenty minutes. When he came out and related all this to me, he was in quite a state of awe. He had other subsequent experiences on different occasions, one involving him asking universal questions in his mind and receiving mind expanding answers. Needless to say, he loved his crystal bed sessions.

I did not have anything so dramatic happen during my crystal bed adventures. But I must say they are other-worldly in their feel, and I felt amazing after each session. You feel totally rejuvenated and full of peace. They are quite the unique experience.

The Waterfall

About a fifteen-minute walk from the Casa is a waterfall that is considered sacred, and one must receive permission from the entities to visit it. It is a beautiful setting, and magical in its appearance. There are rules around dress and the amount of people allowed to go at one time, and I did visit the waterfall a couple of times during my first visit. I did not have anything unusual happen to me during either of my visits, but I am sure on some level I received healing from it, and many speak of miraculous happenings here as well. It is a perfectly joyful experience if only for the fact that it is a cooling balm in an otherwise hot and humid day.

The Current

While I have explained that people line up to go in front of John of God, I will also now explain another of the wonderful healing parts of the whole experience at the Casa. There are three different rooms around the line up that extends to the seat of John of God. They call these current rooms. The energy that is swirling all around the Casa is strong.

The energies coming from the higher realms that work through John of God and collectively in and around the Casa are amazing. You can feel these energies most of the time just by being near the Casa, and even more strongly during the times when John of God is in residence and incorporated.

The entities show up for the scheduled times, but many can be felt at unusual times as well. Anyone wanting to benefit from sitting in the current can show up and sit in the pews in each of the rooms during the morning and afternoon sessions. The first room is for anyone, and it is said to be the strongest current of all. It can be wild in this room because there are lots of people with issues, unbridled emotions and fears sitting here, and the entities are helping all of them. The energy of this room is palpable. As you turn the corner, the second current room faces John of God, and a person must have permission from John of God to sit here. There are also many mediums from all over the world who sit and hold energy and space for the entities to be able to do the miraculous work that they do. These people create and hold a strong positive vibration to keep the high level of energy for healing to be achieved.

The third current is one that offers blessings, balms and peaceful vibrations for people who are in need of such energy. It is the last room where people having been before John of God go to sit and receive energy.

Second to my spiritual operation, my time sitting in the current was the most beneficial time I spent in Abadiana. I had read about the current rooms, and it took me a few days to understand how it all worked and to reap the bounty it had to offer.

I am not the best meditator; it is hard for me to quiet my mind and go to a deep restful place. When a person decides they are going to go sit in the current, you must stay until all people have gone before John of God. This means sitting in one position for about three hours, with your eyes closed. They are very strict around this. It can be quite difficult to settle into this extended mediation.

It was here, in the current, that I had what was probably my most important experience and greatest benefit from my time in Brazil. After the first couple of days, I started to settle into the rhythm of the current. I relaxed into a deep state of quiet in my mind and allowed all my thoughts to drift. All of a sudden, I began to feel pain under my right shoulder blade towards the middle of my back. So I adjusted my posture to relieve this feeling. I could not seem to get comfortable. Again and again I shifted my body trying to get rid of the now excruciating pain.

All of a sudden I had a knowing or awareness that this was not just some random cramp in my body. I knew it was a deeper, more ingrained pain that was buried deep in my cells and wanted to be released. This is what the current can do for a person, the entities will help you bring things up that are deeply ingrained in your subconscious that are really hard to access by yourself. The tricky part was keeping myself focused on this idea, and not giving into the extreme feeling of pain that was threatening to overwhelm me. I find it hard to articulate accurately what I did at this moment, but I will do my best to describe it and hopefully reach you with clarity so that you will be able to use it in your own life.

I reached into my awareness and became someone who was watching the pain. I totally surrendered in this moment at the height of what seemed like more pain than I should have been able to bear. I realized that I would *allow* the pain, I would watch it and not be part of it. I gave in to whatever was going to happen in that moment. Whether I died, whether I lived, whatever was going to happen, I was observing it and content with the outcome, to the point of not caring at all how things went. I intuitively knew that this was what I had to do, and in that eternal moment, the pain was transmuted somehow, it subsided. All of a sudden, I was fine. This was amazing to me, and suddenly my mind took over, I started thinking about this, and marveling at what had just happened. Then it started all over again. I could feel the pain come back, just a little at first, then building in intensity, and finally crescendoing in a full scale octave that was unsustainable to me, and yet again I allowed it, surrendered to it, and once more it was transmuted. After I left the current at the end of the day, I felt great, my shoulder and back felt as if nothing had been bothering them.

When I went back to the current the next day, the same experience happened all over again. This went on for the remainder of the days that I spent in current until I left Brazil. However, each day the pain lessened in intensity, and towards the end of my stay it was there but quite bearable. I realized that I had been shedding some deeply ingrained self-worth issues. I was releasing sadness, grief and pain coming from a multitude of previous lives. This was the gold in my trip to visit John of God and the entities. They were helping me on my path to self-healing, by helping me release the emotional underlying component of my physical illness, and for that I am eternally grateful to them.

I now know and recognize this feeling when it comes up. I have experienced this a few times back here in Canada and know how to surrender to it; I do not need the entities to help me, I just do it on my own. This is why I feel compelled to share this with others—to help them access this on their own, and so affect their own healing, without having to travel all the way to Brazil.

Our visit to John of God was at its end, and my husband and I would find that our time spent there was one of the most magical, healing and peaceful experiences of our lives thus far.

Chapter 22.
SECOND TRIP TO JOHN OF GOD

I felt great after arriving back home. It was the end of the summer, and I was in good spirits after all that had happened in Brazil; I felt I was where I needed to be for now.

I continued to practice all the regular healing methods that had been working for me so far. Diet, supplements, walking, and meditating. I now had more refined skills in allowing my body to be what it wanted to be. I knew how to allow emotional things to come up if they wanted to.

As we moved from summer into late fall, my husband decided he was going to take a trip to western Canada that would have him away for three weeks. He suggested to me that I might benefit from another trip to Brazil and the healing atmosphere that the Casa offers. This came out of the blue, but when I considered his words, I realized that it felt right; I had already made the trip with him and knew where I was going and what the trip entailed. This time I would be there for three whole weeks. By myself! But again, it felt right, so I agreed to go. As always in my travel arrangements, when it is meant to be, it adds up very easily and things unfold seamlessly. This trip was no exception. It unfolded perfectly.

When you are trying to make something happen, and it doesn't unfold easily, then you are usually not meant to go. I listen carefully now to things that do not want to be. An example of this was a cruise I tried to book with certain dates that we wanted, and when I tried to get flights, hotel, etc., none of it would come together. I surrendered and picked different dates, and these plans came together with total ease.

We found out, when we were on the actual cruise, that the dates we had originally tried to get were the worst weather the cruise line had ever experienced. Apparently it was the trip from hell, so we were pretty pleased to not have been on it! The universe always sends you clear messages as to your best path, we just need to listen.

I was not looking forward to the nine-hour overnight flight from Atlanta to Brasilia. The last time we had experienced this flight, we were packed three in a row, in tiny seats, and it was very uncomfortable. Imagine my surprise and pleasure when the last person got on the flight and my row of three seats held only myself. I gave gratitude for this I can assure you. There were two of us who had the three seats to ourselves, the person directly across from me. The rest of the plane was full! Amazing. I lifted up all the armrests, laid down and stretched out, enjoying the almost bed like comfort. This promised to be an awesome trip.

Upon arriving in Brasilia I had no complications getting back into the country. I headed out to the front of the airport to find my connection for my ride to Abadiana. I was booked in once again with the Pousada Luz Divina, and they have their own driver pick up their guests.

As I waited for my luggage, I noticed a blonde woman staring at me. She eventually wandered over and said hello to me and asked where I was staying. I told her and learned she too was staying at the same place, but was going to have to wait until later to arrive as she was meeting her friend, who was coming in on an afternoon flight. I smiled and said I would look forward to seeing her there. I got a feeling that she was a little more intent on me than was normal. Katherine was her name, and her interest would play itself out in time.

Bugs, Bugs, and Things That Crawl In The Night.

Upon arriving in Abadiana, I learned that John of God had been kept a little longer than planned in Italy; he had been out of the country setting up some affiliation in Europe. This is why it is important to book more than one week when going to Brazil, we only booked for one week the first time and had to lengthen our stay at great expense. So for me, being there for three weeks, this was no imposition. I knew that the entities were still around even when John of God was not there, and that one can always participate in the current or enjoy crystal beds.

I was happily tucked into a lovely little room which opened onto a beautiful private garden. I was soon to learn, however, what a difference a few months can make when it comes to changing seasons in Brazil. They were heading into their rainy season, and with this came the bugs.

When we were there in August, it was winter, dry and hot, so very few bugs. Now it was late October and we were entering spring, and with it came blooming trees, and humid wet afternoons and bugs. Have I mentioned the bugs? Canadians are very spoiled in our mostly temperate climate. Nova Scotia has very few issues when it comes to predators. No poisonous snakes and the most annoying bugs are very tiny but respectable mosquitoes and black flies.

I was quite unprepared for the hordes of creepy crawly insects which came out mostly at night, but can also surprise you during the day. My first night was spent sharing my bathroom with an enormous three-inch cockroach. He had himself nicely tucked in under the base of the toilet and would venture out only when the light was out, so I would enter and surprise him, which sent him scurrying back under the toilet. The idea of going to sleep with this large cockroach having free roaming rights in my room, was not something I could live with. I shut the bathroom door, and rolled up a towel and put it tight against the opening along the floor and went to bed and an uneasy sleep. When I got up the next morning, the cockroach was halfway up the wall of my shower, and so I had to endure a shower with him. Kept my eye on him the whole time. Normally when I encounter animals in my life, especially unusual encounters, I look up animal totems and try to figure out what their presence is trying to tell me. So I looked up cockroach and found the following information. *The cockroach teaches us how to use what we have available to us for survival. To clean out the dead and useless aspects of our lives. When the cockroach appears as a totem, our sensitivity to subtle changes will be magnified. We will have the power to scurry out of danger. People with this totem often find that they had an abbreviated childhood—a premature movement into adulthood, the necessity to take on early responsibility. Although often seen as a disgusting animal, the cockroach is actually a gifted teacher in the art of survival and successful adaptability, especially in an environment that may seem a bit hostile.* This actually resonated with me; I was in a strange country by myself, and the change in the season had me a little off. Also, I did lose my mother when I was eight years old and stepped into adulthood almost overnight as a result.

I decided that I had to make my peace with the cockroach, to accept its presence and its right to be there, and to let go of my anxiety and fear of it. It should not have surprised me, but I have to admit that I did not see it again during my entire stay. Making my peace with it dissolved all the energy I was putting out around it—I let go of the resistance. This season proved to be a nightmare for many of the people I met during this time, some of them had so many bugs in their rooms each night that they hardly slept for days, and were pretty stressed overall. I am happy to report that I had a mostly bug-free three weeks, due to my diligence in putting a rolled up towel in front of my door, putting a glass over the drains of both the sink and shower, and keeping the toilet cover down. I released any fears around the bugs and slept great.

I should relate one more bug story, only because it had its humorous side, although not so much for the people on the receiving end. A couple from the UK arrived during my second week and were staying in the room next to mine, called the annex. There were only two rooms in this gorgeous private area. The first night they were there, I was woken up around midnight with the horrific screams of a woman in dire straights. Her husband was yelling and there was much movement and banging going on. I thought to myself, *Ah, the cockroach.* I only found out the following morning that they had had no less than three gigantic centipedes crawling around in their bed! They had gone to sleep and woke up to find them crawling on them.

I was very sympathetic to their plight, and tried to tell them how I was coping. This went on for three nights in a row, for some reason they could not get them out or under control. So the third day the man told me that while his wife was the main reason they were here to see John of God, that she was so stressed that she felt they may have to leave on account of the bugs.

As he told me this, I felt inspired to mention to him to look up the animal totem on the centipedes, as I felt it was interesting that they had the same insect three nights in a row. I did not know how this information would be received, one is never sure of the level of awareness and receptivity some people have, but I felt it might help and I did want to see them move through this and have a calmer experience here at the Casa. I told him to go online and read a few different versions of the animal totem to get a rounded view, and then see if there was a message that made sense to them and their particular lives and situation.

Later that day he came up to me and said it was ironic how much the animal totem resonated with them. As a result, they did not have any repeat visitations, and all was quiet for the duration of their stay. However, he did still seem to attract some interesting characters. One night I was coming into the compound that housed our rooms as it was getting quite dark, and he asked me if I wanted to come over and see the enormous tarantula he had almost just stepped on. I replied in the negative, I did not need to have any visuals before going to a sleep that would not send me off to a happy place.

Significant Meetings

The following day while having lunch, I met the woman from the airport again. She and her male friend from Scotland had arrived and we exchanged names. Upon meeting her male friend, I had an instant feeling of recognition on some level of this person. I had not felt that way with Katherine, but did feel something under the surface with David, her friend.. These two people were to become very good friends for the duration of my stay.

I very much enjoyed my time with Katherine as I got to know her, and it would be through her that I would eventually learn of the scalar energy pendant. There was an overarching feeling between the three of us that there were deeper connections at play. Katherine at one point revealed to me that she had experienced a feeling around me when I first got onto the airplane—she felt she *knew* me.

They proved to be interesting companions, and we shared many threads of knowledge and stories during our time in Brazil. I still keep in contact with both of them, although with time and distance, it has diminished somewhat. After I arrived back home in Nova Scotia, I had a dream that I was on the planet *Niburu* with both Katherine and David. At the time of the dream I had no idea what Niburu was. I had to look it up online, and it is a planet that intersects with Earth's orbit every 3,600 years. So I decided to ask the entity Veronica about this dream. She told me that I was living a life on Niburu right now as well, and that these two people were both in that life with me. I love it when I have dreams that reveal to me what I am doing in other dimensions, places and times.

The Current (Again)

During my second trip, I was excited to get back to the current, now that I knew what it entailed and understood the benefits of sitting in it. I knew that I still had emotional stuff to release, and so I set about doing just that.

The first day I again had the pain come up in my shoulder area, into my back a bit, and down my arms. It was not as bad as the first time, but substantial enough. During the three days of the first week it got less and less and finally by the end of the week I could sit in the current with ease and enjoy the long meditation it afforded.

John of God (Again)

The second week, John of God was back and so, on the Wednesday morning, all of us excitedly herded down to the Casa. It is quite a sight watching hundreds of people walk down a small quiet street in South America all wearing white. It is kind of cultish looking, and my husband I had watched ourselves take part in this ritual with quite a sense of humor around it the first time. We laughed with each other as we pondered what most of our North American family and friends would think if they could see us participating in this experience. Not that we cared, but one did have to see the humor in it. After all, this was tame compared to our experiences in the Philippines.

I lined up with everyone and had my question ready, and again the first thing I was told: "Operation this afternoon." You get a mixed feeling when you are told this, as you want to get the most help they can give you while you are there, and if you need an operation, then it is necessary, but no one really looks forward to the twenty-four-hour solitary confinement. This time, however, I was more prepared for the whole experience and was determined to pay attention to the subtleties that came with it. The first time I did not know what to expect, but this time I was ready to be more present around what actually transpires in each moment.

Second Spiritual Operation

My operation this time was much different. First of all, I felt very peaceful and surrendered while it was going on. I did not really feel much during the actual operation this time, but felt very tired and spaced out after it was finished. However, when I got back to my room and got into bed, I felt like I was floating and in a state of euphoria for about four hours. I was totally awake but could feel electric pulses all over my body and could feel them more specifically in my breast and stomach area. At one time I felt stinging pains all around my abdomen. Overlying all of this was a feeling of supreme nurturing and peaceful happiness. Very different from my first experience. I was also in a state of total acceptance and gratitude this time around, which certainly made for a more noticeable experience. This was followed by quite a few intense and revealing dreams, which would need another book to go into!

Codes and Keys

In addition to my new found friends Katherine and David, I also met a beautiful woman from New Zealand named Glenice. We eventually were rounded out by the inclusion of one of the young mediums living at the Casa, whom I had met during my first trip. Her name was Irini. This was to be a time of friendship, a magical coming together of souls whom I know I have interacted with many times during various incarnations. I now understand that this time of sharing experiences and conversations with this group was an unlocking of what are considered codes and keys within a person's blueprint. The soul's plan for all of existence is contained in the blueprint. All interactions are timed so as to unlock the next levels or shifts of experience and expansion. I was to learn much more about codes, keys and blueprints from a guide who would come to me at the appropriate time for the unlocking of our codes.

We became a close group for the three weeks I was there, always coming together for lunch and supper and talking amongst ourselves late into the evening. There seemed to be a need to be together, and I felt that Irini was serving a special service to us all in her presence, as she is quite gifted in her abilities to communicate with guides and angels and all such spirit entities. Her role at the Casa was to help the entities come through easier; she held the light through her amazing singing ability. She always seemed to have one foot in the material world and another in the higher realms. A beautiful soul. And so we wound our way through many thoughts, questions and ideas about what and who we were here to be, and I know much was served in our souls and our individual healing by these interactions.

Glenice and David were particularly entertaining—he was a young man from Scotland with an acerbic sense of humor, and Glenice was a gentle but racy kiwi (from New Zealand), and the clash of their individual sense of humor created great fun for the rest of us.

Irini especially loved their fun and play. At different points during the three weeks, Irini was to give each of us a specific gift that she was guided to give to us. Mine was an amethyst crystal that she was guided to give to me by Archangel Michael. She gave this to me just prior to my having my operation. I felt very excited to be given this, and placed it next to my heart as I was having the actual operation.

I actually met Irini for the first time during my initial visit to Brazil. We had asked Irini if she could give us toning lessons. My husband had suggested that we could benefit from such a thing after reading something in a book around the benefits of toning for the chakras.

Serendipitously, that very same day, a woman mentioned to us that there was a young woman who gave singing lessons to the locals to make some money on the side. Bob looked at me meaningfully and we tracked her down. I was to learn she had a beautiful pitch perfect voice.

One of the stringent rules at the Casa is that no one is to receive any other healing while undergoing your time with the entities. They do not want any conflicting energy interfering with their efforts for you. So Irini told us she would have to ask the entities if she could do this. She asked, and received a yes, and so we went to her house one beautiful afternoon. It's pretty much a beautiful afternoon every day in Brazil except during the rainy season.

She led us outside underneath a lush mango tree, and there proceeded to take us through the tonal sounds of our chakras. During this, she was guided to do some things that were unexpected by all of us. At one point she guided my husband to put his arms around me and to sing the word *shema* a certain number of times. During this my husband had a vision of my eye with a large tear rolling down from it. Irini commented to him afterwards that, yes, she could see the deep pain and sadness in my heart.

At the end of the whole experience, she asked us to give gratitude to the entities that had been present with us helping. She stated that the energies of Archangel Michael, Mother Mary and Dr. Augusta had all been there.

This was very intriguing to me, as my logical mind still always wanted linear proof around such experiences, and this synchronicity provided it. Irini could not have known who had performed my initial operation the first time, as I had not yet met her. I only knew that Dr. Augusta had performed my surgery due to my guide Ananda having chatted with the volunteer who interprets for John of God, telling her who was present during that operation. So I felt very loved and serene around this wonderful experience.

The rest of my visit in Brazil was spent mostly allowing myself to heal in the peacefulness and heat of the village, while sharing many stories and threads of information with our small group.

I did have one very enlightening talk with Irini before leaving. She made a point of seeking me out one day to impart to me that she was guided to tell me that she could see very clearly that I was a being of light, and that I should stop undervaluing myself. She said that just because I do not get visions does not mean that I am not being clearly guided. I could hear the truth of what she was saying to me.

I have always wished to have more immediate experiences, such as visions, or audible connections with spirit. And I realize I am very well-guided, just in a way that requires me to trust my higher self. This is part of my chosen experience at this time, and I appreciated her telling me this truth. It was very valuable to me. And so ended my second trip to Brazil and John of God. I would highly recommend this trip to anyone who can manage to travel there, regardless of whether your desire is to obtain some form of healing or to just enhance your own spiritual path. The energies there are magnificent, peaceful, loving and pure. My eternal gratitude to them all.

Oprah and John of God

Almost a year after I left Brazil, Oprah did a show on John of God. There was an initial story run in her magazine "O", experienced and written by one of her television show producers. This woman felt a desire to go to Brazil based on the death of her father and found great solace and healing as a result of visiting with John of God. Oprah herself went to experience the energy at the spiritual hospital in Brazil, and taped a full show documenting the amazing benefits of the site. Included in the show was an in-depth interview with John of God. You can access the full version online.

Orbs

My husband and I were unaware of *orbs* until our trip to Brazil. For anyone wanting to see what orbs look like, just Google the term "pictures orbs", and you will see many varieties and colors of them. Often people will see them only when using a camera, they will show up in a picture in close proximity to someone.

We were walking home from the Casa one evening and happened upon a photographer from France taking random pictures of the black night sky. Being curious as to what he could possibly be doing, we approached him and asked. He told us he was trying to get various pictures of orbs. He explained to us that he would take a picture of a piece of night sky and it would show a couple of orbs when he looked at the taken shot. Then he would take the same shot of the same night sky just seconds later and get hundreds of orbs. This was baffling to him. We all ventured out one night with our cameras and took various shots of orbs. All of us pointed our cameras at the same piece of sky. One of our group got one shot with the whole frame literally peppered with them. Another person noted that she got more when she sang.

My husband did not fair that well overall; the French photographer laughingly told him they did not like Kodak cameras! They do not appear to conform to the current laws of known physics, or time and space as we currently understand it. There is not a lot of definitive information on what orbs actually are, but many theories abound. I feel that they are groupings of energies of light that are of similar purpose or intent in their adding to the fabric of creation. The great proliferation of them at the Casa is almost surely connected in some way with help given to so many people by the entities that are found there.

Chapter 23.
CRYSTALS

The awareness and value of the healing aspects of crystals was starting to come to me prior to my trip to the Philippines. However, after being in Brazil and realizing the amazing properties and sentient abilities that crystals hold, they have become quite a wonderful complement to my healing regime. They actually started to find me!

Just prior to my trip to Brazil, during one of my reiki sessions with Elizabeth, she mentioned to me that she had been shown an amazing piece of snow white quartz crystal very close to where I live. It lies right along a stretch of beautiful beach on the Atlantic Ocean. It is quite large, and I was astounded by it when I went to see it. She told me that she had sat on it and had felt quite a *buzz* from it. She felt it would be beneficial for me to lay on it and get the healing energies from the crystal. It sticks up out of the ground for a length of about twenty to thirty feet and is about ten feet wide. That is just the tip of it. There are places all around the area where little bits of it are poking through to the surface. So it is quite a big concentration of quartz in that area and goes very deep into the earth. Nova Scotia in general is quite well known for its quantity of snow or milky quartz. Milky quartz is known to possess *feminine energy* or *moon energy* as opposed to clear quartz, which possesses *masculine energy*, or *sun energy*.

I had a very interesting experience, one that definitely falls into the area of synchronicity around my first visit to the snow quartz at the beach. I laid on it for an hour and watched the beautiful waves move in an out in rhythmic fashion. Very peaceful. Then I felt an overwhelming desire to have a piece of this crystal to take home with me. However, none of it wanted to yield to me easily, and I did not feel right hacking away at it—like some people had obviously done.

The very next day I went back again to enjoy another peaceful healing hour on the quartz plateau. Beside this piece of quartz, the province had placed a park bench. As I arrived I noticed three large and very different shaped pieces of snow quartz sitting on the bench. One was smaller and triangular, with a very smooth bottom. The second was round and polished like a beach stone, but entirely filled the palm of my hand. The third was the most interesting of all: it had a face carved into it. Very obviously a face, anyone who has seen it since, sees the face immediately. It resembles my husband I might add. I am just being truthful here. It really does. Needless to say I was pretty excited! But then I had the thought that they must be someone else's crystals. That someone had found them on the beach and had left them there while they walked, or something like that.

I stayed for my hour, and at the end, since no one had claimed them, I felt surely that they had been left for me. What are the odds of having three such pieces—that I had so fervently desired the previous day—sitting there waiting for me. Perfection. I have had interesting experiences and dreams with these crystals, and they were my first experience with the amazing abilities that crystals hold. Crystals are alive and a means of communication with other realms of existence.

The spiritual hospital in Brazil is built on a plateau overlaying a bed of quartz crystal. Brazil is one of the richest countries in the world in terms of sheer quantity and quality of quartz crystals—and gemstones in general. The night sky actually shimmers from the dust of the crystals in the air.

We noticed one night at the Casa, when we were taking pictures of orbs, that when the flash went off from our cameras, the air shimmered like reflections of diamond dust. We were mesmerized with this magical experience. It never got old.

It is no coincidence that the entities guided John of God to build his spiritual hospital in this precise location, for the sheer amount of crystal allows the entities to better do their work. There are tons of crystals for sale at the Casa, for a mere fraction of the price charged elsewhere in the world. They are also enhanced with the focused energies of the entities. My husband and I brought back many crystals from Brazil.

I now wear crystals at all times on my body. I have them in my house—more specifically all around my bedroom. I have many right beside my bed, and I always sleep with one. Transformation to higher awareness is much accelerated with the presence of crystals. I have added below some very good information around crystals for the enhanced awareness of the reader from sources that are a bit more knowledgeable than I around the totality of their amazing abilities. I love my crystals.

> *How do Crystals work for and with you? In a much oversimplified explanation, the energy radiating from Quartz Crystals naturally resonates at the quantum level in harmony with human (and other) frequencies - in other words in harmony with human energy speeds. In this context, "resonates" means it reinforces naturally occurring oscillations because the frequency of the Crystal is the same as the frequency of its source - the primal life force energy.*

> *Naturally terminated Crystals are synchronized, are automatically "in alignment" with, the original cosmic energy. In other words, Quartz Crystals are just naturally in harmony with the life force in its raw still unformed state. The precise internal arrangement of Quartz Crystals ensures this constant and consistent harmony - your Crystals literally help you stay in tune, when you let them.*

> *This is why holding a Crystal, meditating with one, carrying or sleeping with one, or just having them around works*

so well. Your Crystals continually and with virtually no effort on your part try their best to keep you in tune with their own natural harmonic synchronization with the life force energy - they naturally try their best to keep you in harmony with life. And since each Crystal is a distinct individual with its own harmonic frequency, yes, it can, make a difference which one you use when. Sometimes you need an energy booster, sometimes a tranquilizer.

The human body is, among other things, a big receiving instrument. It has even developed specialized parts to receive and then translate certain frequencies so they "make sense" to us - we call these parts eyes, ears, skin, etc. Using this analogy, your brain is the tuner and your nervous system the antennae. Crystals, then, can function as your satellite dish, radar, internet networks, links, plug-ins - you get the idea. They extend, enhance, and amplify your own natural abilities. In fact the primary function of Quartz Crystal is to boost and amplify energy.

So when you hold a Crystal for even a brief second, it begins to vibrate on a frequency in harmony with your physical body. Remember that it's already resonating with the primal life force energy. Think of Crystals as members of a band or choir - different Crystals contribute their own sounds (frequencies) - not the same notes you're playing, but harmonizing notes - which naturally boost, amplify, align your own. Just one reason why you feel better carrying or wearing one Crystal one day and another the next.

Crystals don't actually hold electrical charges of energy the way a batter can (although they can store other kinds of energy.) But individual Crystals when rubbed or squeezed do produce an electrical charge called piezoelectricity - piezo just means applied pressure. This is the talent of Quartz that has made it the darling of the technological crowd. Crystals are in fact so effective in various technologies that they are now grown in environmentally-controlled labs to ensure that their internal structures are absolutely perfect.

While Crystals are great conductors of almost any type of energy, they're really lousy at conducting heat and cold. This is the reason why Crystals should never be exposed to rapid changes in temperatures. Don't put a cold one in hot water or a warm one in ice water, or leave them in your car or window on really hot or cold days for example. And please, please don't put them in your freezer. Yeah, people do that - and often end up with cracked or shattered stones later. Trapped air and gas freezes and thaws first...and then boom.

On that note, chipped or otherwise imperfect Crystals don't necessarily lose their qualities. They don't have to be perfect (which often translates to expensive) to do their thing. We call these damaged ones Warrior and Empathic Crystals, depending on the damage, and have found them great reminders that getting some very rough and unfair treatment doesn't make us less. Often it's the chips and wounds that create the appearance of the rainbow in the Crystal - making a Warrior or an Empath are excellent reminders that we have the internal power to do the same, no matter how we look to outsiders.

Crystal energy frequencies also have the inherent ability to give you support when you're trying to dig information out of your subconscious - information you know at some level but stuff you're not consciously aware of at the moment for one reason or another.

[Excerpted in part from Crystal Personalities: A Quick Reference to Special Forms of Quartz]

Chapter 24.
VISIONS

As I previously stated, I have always been intrigued and somewhat envious of people whose abilities involve visions, those who are clairvoyant and/or clairaudient. This seems so straightforward—you see something or you hear something—clear and direct experience. I have the *gift of knowing*. This means that I just know things. I get a feeling or a thought that tells me something is important or an answer to something just pops into my head, and I have a 100% knowing that it is true or important. I have learned to listen to these. So imagine my happiness and surprise when I finally received a vision. In actual fact, I received two. Both were during my second trip to Brazil.

My first vision came to me during the night when I woke up at 1:11 and deciding that this being an auspicious time and all, I would ask out loud for assistance in connecting more immediately with the divine feminine energy. I had no sooner voiced this than I had a flash inside my mind of a picture of an antique key ring with four keys on it. I can clearly see it to this day, it was very precise and intricate. I was ecstatic to be given this, even though I still do not know the absolute meaning of it, I did find out that silver keys are related to feminine energy and the moon.

The second vision came on my flight home. I had just laid my head against the window of the airplane and closed my eyes. I was awake but quite relaxed. And, clear as day, I had a picture shown to me of a large stone wall—sandstone it looked to be—and carved into the stone was the word *Isnofret*. That was it. Very clear, but what did it mean?

My first inclination was that it was an Egyptian word, and so upon arriving home, I Googled it, but all that came up was Isetnofret, or Asetnofret, each a different spelling of the name of the second wife of Pharaoh Ramses II. So I felt that it must be related to this. During my next conversation with the entity Veronica, I decided to ask her about this vision. She replied to me: "I know you think this is from an ancient language, but it is actually from an 'ancient, ancient' language, from Lemuria, and it means Victory." She sounded very pleased as she said this to me. Needless to say, I was very excited to hear this. Victory in whatever form it comes is welcome.

There is a distinction between imagination, dreams, and visions. I now know the difference between all three of these, as all of us can imagine things, and I get very prophetic and clear dreams at times, but the visions were very direct and totally different from the other two experiences.

Chapter 25.
SCALAR ENERGY

I was now back in Nova Scotia, heading towards the Christmas Season, and coming down off my beautiful energy from Brazil. Most people who have been to the Casa of John of God, always remark on how much of a difference they notice in the harmony of their energy fields after leaving the warm and peaceful frequency of the Casa. Coming back into the real world of mass consciousness after that experience, I could strongly feel a difference in density! It's like going from a soft feather bed to a hardwood floor.

During this time, I had some very interesting things come forward. One of them was around *scalar energy*, a term I had never before heard.

First it came in the form of an email from Katherine, the lady I had met in Brazil. She sent me an article on scalar energy and something called a *rife machine*, technology involving zero-point energy developed by Nikola Tesla—a very important and amazing man who had been involved in trying to bring free energy to the planet during the late 1800s.

Katherine felt that such a thing would be beneficial to me in helping to heal my cancer. So I read all about it that first afternoon and mentioned it to my husband, who also read the information. As a result we read about other modalities of the same technology called scalar energy pendants. The very next day, out of left field, I received a call from my sister-in-law. I do not stay in close contact with this particular family member, so it was a bit unusual to get a call from her. And more unusual was her question to me. She wanted to know if I wanted a scalar energy pendant? She did not even know what it was, but had been telling one of her uncles about my situation, and he offered it to her for me; he had gotten it for someone else, who was not using it, and felt it could be beneficial for me. Astounding! What are the odds of two such occurrences around such an obscure technology happening a day apart? Such synchronicity is not to be ignored! So I told her YES, I would love to have it, and have worn it around my neck ever since.

Simply put, scalar energy ups the level of frequency that your cells vibrate at. Diseased cells vibrate lower than healthy cells. I had read various reports from people who wear scalar energy pendants, and their experiences when first putting them on. Some hardly noticed a change; others said they had to take them off at bedtime, as they interfered with their ability to get to sleep. All I can say is that, for myself, I did notice for the first couple of hours after I put it on that I felt like I had had five cups of coffee—I have not drank coffee for years. Since that initial feeling, I have been fine. I do not notice any difference when I take it off or put it back on. I generally do not sleep with mine on. I did take the opportunity to ask Veronica about it, however; and she laughed saying: "It is not doing what you think it is doing, but it is helping, so keep it on." There is not always a complete linear understanding of the answers Veronica gives at certain times, but I just accepted the validation that it was helping and feels right. You can do your own research around scalar energy and decide for yourself if you feel it would be right for you.

Another interesting thing happened around this time, one which could be taken as a combined dream/vision. I had been speaking at length with one of my daughters about her desire to bring forward more scientific information around the energy field of the body. She has taken a degree in biology and also philosophy with the overall intention of moving into bio-ethics, and has a great interest in the energy body.

It is very difficult to bring forward theories in the metaphysical arena within a university setting, so she is always walking a fine line and has to have strong provable scientific formulas for her ideas. She stated to me during a conversation we were having one day that she wished she had some way of visibly showing the auric field around a body.

I didn't give this much thought really, and so was surprised at the dream I had two nights later. In the dream I was shown two words, *Kirlian effect*. Very front and center in my visual field, almost like they were large words hanging in the sky. I even remember thinking in the dream, it's a good thing they spelled it, because if I had heard these words, I would have spelled the first word with a C.

I felt very strongly that this was important, as I woke up in the middle of the night and had to tell myself a couple of times to remember it in the morning. As it turned out, I almost did forget about it. But it came to me again, and I realized I had better Google it and see what it meant.

Imagine my delight when I found out that Kirlian photography is a specific form of photography that takes pictures of the energy displayed around any living form. This includes humans, plants, animals, etc. It is very expensive, but totally scientific. This is a very good example of how I trust what I get in dreams. We hold all knowledge within us, and only need to ask and then get out of the way to receive.

Chapter 26.

DOROTHY

I have a lovely friend, Drita, who is originally from Albania. Drita is a reiki master, and is extremely committed to healing all those who come her way. You can view Drita's site online at www.selfinlove.com. She is someone who came into my life at exactly the right time—as is the way of the universe.

In her continuing self-discovery as a healer, she had been taking some online courses from a woman named Dorothy who lived in New Zealand. Now Dorothy is quite an amazing healer in her own right as I was to find out. Drita decided to invite her to come to Canada and stay with her while she received her training.

When I came back from Brazil, I received a couple of calls from Drita encouraging me to come and see Dorothy for a healing session. By this time, I had done quite a lot towards my healing and really wanted to coast for a bit and let myself recover from my efforts thus far. I put her request in the back of my mind and left it there.

About a month before Dorothy was scheduled to head back to New Zealand, I received another call from Drita, again asking me to please come and see her. This coincided with my regular call to Veronica, and so it was while I had only a couple of minutes left in my call, that I was suddenly inspired to ask Veronica about Dorothy. I always ask Veronica to give me their view on the level of ability of all the healers I engage with.

I have found this to be of great benefit, as not all healers that come my way get high points from Veronica. Dorothy was one who did. I barely got the request out of my mouth when they stated vigorously:"Yes, she is a profound healer!"So I called Drita and booked a session. It was to be a great experience.

Dorothy was not quite what I was expecting. She had black hair, piercing blue eyes, and exuded health and vitality. She was also very direct and pleasant with a confidence that many would find overwhelming. I, however, love confident people. You could tell that she lives in her truth and cares not a whit for what anyone thinks of her. She is a woman very grounded in her own abilities and her purpose and passion for being on this earth. Like me, she loves to talk. I also liked to listen to her.

She had much to impart that was of supreme interest to me. She works much like any reiki practitioner does, working with the energy and facilitating the movement of it. The difference is that Dorothy sees the energy with her third eye, can see the colors of the aura, the sacred geometry, the language of light. She can also see what would be considered other worldly things, like people who show up from other time lines, which could be an aspect of a person from a past or future life, along with energies that would be termed aliens.

I had three hands on sessions with her before she left, and all three were awesome experiences. During the first one she had a look at my energy and proceeded to work her magic. At the end of it, I felt amazingly good—as a person always does when receiving reiki from someone who is genuinely gifted with this ability—and she told me what she had seen.

The first time, a woman showed up from around the sixteenth century and just stood at my head and watched what was going on. Dorothy did not know who she was, but she had a feeling it was me from a life during that time. She felt she was connected to my current situation in some sort of way. This woman did not try to help in any way, just observed.

The second visit was a bit more interesting. During this one she told me that the woman showed up right at the beginning—again just observing—but then as she was doing the healing an *Arcturian* (a sixth dimensional being from the planet Arcturus, well regarded in the universe for their advanced healing technologies) showed up to help amplify Dorothy's efforts on my behalf. She said the woman could not get out of there fast enough when the Arcturian showed up.

You can imagine this was quite interesting to me. I often laugh to myself as I consider all the different experiences and stories I am guided to share with everyone, as I do realize how unusual my stories appears to others as they read it. Courage is needed to operate *outside the box* of ordinary everyday limited thought. Dorothy had this in spades. A beautiful mentor for me. She also mentioned that I should be grateful to have such high-priced extraterrestrial help looking out for me. And I am.

My third and last visit was just as fascinating. At the end of it, Dorothy shared a story with me about her own journey. She told me that, at one point in her life, she had recall of a life she lived in Egypt where she was the head of an order of priestesses. During a particular ritual/ceremony she held a staff which had a large crystal at the top of it. She grounded the staff and, at this point, a large white snake was released from it. She told me that was the only time she has ever seen the white snake in her lifetime. She then added that, during my healing session, the white snake appeared above my crown, and then took its fangs and sunk them into my left breast. She said the more interesting thing was that *she* had not called the white snake, I had.

There are not many references to white snakes, but it's most accepted symbolism is that of *kundalini energy*, which is considered to be the creative sexual energy of the divine feminine. The movement of the kundalini of the earth is symbolized by the white snake.

My particular cancer in the breast is associated emotionally with unresolved sexual abuse and unworthiness. The white snake has come to me in dreams as well. Also once in a book about Atlantis. So I felt the importance of this particular healing session. She also told me that she could see where energy goes, and that I had nothing to worry about; I was going to be on the planet for a while yet. I loved my time with Dorothy, and I am grateful to her for our shared experiences. You can find more information about Dorothy and her healing modalities at www.energytherapies.com.

Chapter 27.
EXTRATERRESTRIAL ENERGIES

Because I mentioned alien energies, I would like to comment and expand on information regarding this subject. Some of Dorothy's published books talk about her experience with off world energies.

This is a very controversial subject. Many people believe in the presence of extraterrestrials, and much is both hinted at and ridiculed when it comes to this subject. I would like to offer some information that I have been made aware of where people can do some research and make up their own minds. Of course, by now you know that I believe in such things. I have my own personal experiences to lend weight to this.

As I have stated before, I have quite prophetic dreams at times and have learned to trust what I am getting from my dreams as forms of awareness and guidance. I have dreamt of myself in different form, on other planets, and have seen myself and others as alien beings—some of them reptilian. It is quite an interesting experience I can tell you, and not what you would imagine it to be like at all. The other beings I am conversing with in the dreams seem very natural to me in that state. It is about being not afraid to have esoteric thoughts and having an open mind when it comes to new ideas and concepts that transcend ways in which we have been taught to think on this planet. It is time to open up to new worlds and new meetings. I love the excitement of this. It feels very natural to me.

Keep in mind as you read on that, just like everything in a polarity universe, there are benevolent alien energies, and what we would term not so benevolent energies. Some aliens are here at this time for their own purposes and others are helping out humanity in this time of great awakening. It is helpful to remember that all incarnated souls, whether they are on planet earth or elsewhere, create their own reality, and so no interaction that is ever experienced is done so against a soul's will. All parties agree to the experience for the sake of soul evolvement.

My first serious awareness around extra terrestrials came to me years ago while I was sitting in my doctor's office awaiting my visit with her. I picked up an issue of *Time* magazine, and on the cover was a headline story about a Harvard Professor of Psychiatry named John E. Mack.

This man went on to describe how he felt compelled to come forward after years of listening to hundreds of accounts of the same phenomena about alien abduction from people who were considered to be mentally unstable as a result of their tales. All of the stories given to him by individuals were remarkably similar, even though many of them lived thousands of miles from each other, and often in different countries.

Included in the article were many drawings from these unrelated individuals, all with hauntingly familiar graphic pictures of alien beings and experiences. I was quite moved by this, and like other times in my life, I knew that it was important that I was being shown this information in such a random way. I stored it in my mind and let it go for the time being.

It was only recently, as I was starting to write this book, that I remembered this man. And while I could not find the *Time* magazine article online—a curious detail—I did find copious amounts of information on John Mack.

This man was ridiculed by many and was investigated by Harvard because of his beliefs, even though all his research was done while being employed by Harvard. He spent many years trying to bring this information forward to the public in a credible way. He was killed by a drunk driver in 2004, but his legacy is only starting to come to the forefront.

He is now considered to be the most important scientist ever to dare to admit the truth about the abduction phenomena.

Vanity Fair published an article on him in May of 2013, chronicling his amazing feats as a Pulitzer Prize-winning biographer, and Harvard Medical School Psychiatrist, who was diligent in speaking his truth about his conclusions.

On the Oprah Winfrey show in the 1990s, Mack stated:"Every other culture in history, except this one, in the history of the human race, has believed there were other entities, other intelligences in the universe. Why do we treat people like they're crazy, humiliate them, if they're experiencing some other intelligence?"The majority of people who claimed to be abducted also said that the encounters, while disturbing on some levels, also richly enhanced their lives.This Oprah show can be viewed on YouTube in its entirety.

Also mentioned in the *Vanity Fair* article is the news that Make Magic Productions and Robert Redford's Wildwood Enterprises are making a feature film about John Mack. He has published numerous articles, written books, and spoken at many conferences.You can view more on this courageous man by going to his site at www.johnemackinstitute.org.

The second site I would suggest people view, if they are seeking credible information on UFOs and extraterrestrials, is www.citizenhearing.org. This site chronicles an event called The Citizen Hearing on Disclosure. From April 29, 2013, to May 3, 2013, researchers, activists, political leaders and military agency witnesses representing ten countries gave testimony in Washington DC to six former members of the United States Congress on the evidence for an extraterrestrial presence engaging the human race.With over thirty hours of testimony from forty witnesses over five days, the event was the most concentrated body of evidence regarding the extraterrestrial issue ever presented to the press and the general public at one time. The hearing was also broadcast live over the internet.

I watched quite a lot of this event online myself and was very intrigued by the integrity of the witnesses themselves. Paul Hellyer, an ex-Defense Minister of Canada, spoke of his knowledge of aliens.Apollo veteran astronaut Edgar Mitchell also spoke of his knowledge of alien engagement within the government. They are but two of a long list of credible people who gave testimony. The essence of this testimony is that there is quite a long history of governments worldwide engaging in interactions with certain alien groups and keeping this information from the masses. A truth embargo so to speak. This disclosure movement is asking for the lies to stop and to recognize the massive amount of credible witnesses worldwide who have experienced the alien presence.

Chapter 28.

LAURA

The year 2010 came to an end, and I entered 2011 fully grounded in my approach to life and my continuing journey to total health. I felt I had finished with the need to have such immediate and intense healing such as what I had received from Jun Labo and John of God. I felt that I had the direction of my healing firmly in hand and could progress now on my own and felt very secure in this feeling.

There is a saying that goes *when the student is ready, the teacher shows up*. And so Laura entered my life. She would prove to be a wonderful, enlightened, pure and loving guide for me. It would also be the hardest, most confusing time of my life. And so I begin the tale of my journey with Laura.

It started with yoga. I had always held a fascination and underlying desire to take up yoga. I had been aware of it in the early seventies, while attending a fitness club at that time, I saw some people performing the poses. It was always in the back of my mind to take up yoga at some point in my life.

I signed up for a local class in my small village about five years ago. The teacher was a very interesting woman, and upon reflection, I do believe the reason I attended the class was to hear her message and then remember it when my own time came. You see, she started the class by telling us that she had been diagnosed with uterine cancer about six years previous. She was not given much hope around her outcome from the doctors. So she decided that she would go home and go back to doing yoga. She had always practiced it, and for some reason had stopped. She cleared her mind of any fear around her cancer, lived in the moment, and she is still here today. This was impressed upon my mind at the time. I admired her conviction. Her type of yoga did not really appeal to me overall, and so I did not go back.

As I moved into the New Year of 2011, I decided that the time had come to make yoga a serious part of my healing regime. My husband worked with a woman who went to a yoga class every day at lunchtime. I would often chat with this woman about my unfolding healing journey and all the things I was learning about higher consciousness, spirituality, and the universe at large. She held similar interests. She would often remark to me:

"You should meet my yoga teacher, Laura."

One day in early February, I told her I was ready to meet her friend the yoga instructor. I started with a morning class, twice a week. Now Laura, as I would soon discover in spades, was not like ordinary yoga instructors. Nor was she like ordinary people—period! This was to be a time of unveiling and self-discovery on a level I could never have imagined. I would not have missed it for the world. I can say that now.

My first impression of Laura from my initial yoga class was one of sincere welcoming. She made me feel at home in her small private studio. At this point she only ever had a maximum of five students at any one time. She guided me through all the moves that others were doing during this class and told me just to do them to the best of my ability. She kept a watchful eye on my every move, and quickly corrected me if I was not doing it right, in a very mild way. She explained the importance of the benefits of being in the pose correctly. She always ended her class with a fifteen minute guided meditation. Like the others, I found this to be the best part of the whole experience. Laura has been gifted with a most beautiful and unusual voice, one that calms and soothes a person's emotional body. As I was to learn, she has an energy around her that makes everyone feel wonderful to be in her presence.

Atlantis

Around my third yoga class, as I was preparing to leave, Laura started talking to me. "I know you," she said. "I know you from Atlantis. I can see the tall headpiece you wore there; it is around your head now." I was listening to her and trying to come to terms with what she was saying. She seemed compelled and at the same time somewhat reluctant to be saying what she was saying. I could see her dilemma. She worried that I would not hear or not understand; nonetheless, she felt compelled to share this. And so began the phase of our time together that was to transcend yoga.

It started with Atlantis. This is what she told me at this time about herself and about me and about Atlantis. She said that we were sisters in Atlantis at the time of its fall and that I was a political leader of some sort, one who oversaw many factions of leadership, and that she had a healing centre there, where she used crystals. She said that I had brought a crystal to her then for coding for this time. She explained to me that she is what is known as a walk in, which is an energy that comes into an already existing body when the soul of that body dies/departs. There is always an agreement between both the outgoing and incoming soul around this exchange.

She said she remembered coming from Andromeda as light into the body. She knew she had to live out the karma of the girl's body she was in until such time as the soul contract was completed. Then she would have the use of the body for her own destiny here on the planet. This completion ended about a week before I met her for the first time.

She told me that she had always been shown that she would heal someone with breast cancer, and so was not surprised when she first met me. She was made aware of our meeting very shortly before my coming to her yoga studio by feeling pain and a lump in her own breast—that was the energy showing her that it wanted attention. She told it to leave and awaited the unfolding of our meeting.

She recognized me immediately as the person she had been waiting for. I was to learn later from her about codes and blueprints and how they are unlocked as a result of seemingly chance meetings which are really the overall planned coming together at the appropriate time. Energy revealing itself. This was just such an example: the codes for both of us were unlocked and so we could move forward with the next level of experience.

Imagine my excitement and skepticism around all I had been told by her. I was not quite sure what to do about this. I felt very sure that there was something there, it felt right. But I also was still very much in my logical mind as well. I still allowed my mind to intrude and question much of the time. It is a progression to quiet the mind and trust the heart. So be kind to yourselves as you move through the transition. I can say this with hindsight! I pondered how much of this I was to trust and move into the energy of. So I did what I usually do when I am not quite sure of how to proceed in matters outside of the linear physical world: I called Veronica. In time I would learn to trust Laura and all that she knows and reveals, but at this time I still needed my guidance from Veronica.

I had learned to trust the guidance I receive from Veronica. They have never steered me wrong on the big issues such as my health; however, it can be a bit more taxing trying to understand the large overarching scope of the multidimensional aspects of my time here on earth in this incarnation.

Unsure as to what was unfolding here, I asked them about Laura—I gave them the name Laura and asked how she was connected to me. That is all I said to them. This is the wonder and amazement I still hold around these nonphysical entities. Their unfailing ability to give you such succinct and personal information from just a name. Names are frequency, and as such they can see the energy of the frequency of the name you give them. They have the ability to delve into what is called the *Akashic Records* which hold all thoughts and experiences of every soul on the planet for all of their incarnations.

They told me that she was a person who was in the multidimensional realms the majority of the time, that she was a clear energy, a light being, and that she and I had created a vortex of energy from the time of Atlantis to this particular time period. So I then asked if I was a priestess during this time. They laughed and said that would be a junior version of who I was then, that I was a leader of many groups in Atlantis and that I had an advanced healing experience during that life. This lent quite a lot of credibility to Laura's claims, to say the least. Two versions, both saying the same thing. At this point Laura had never heard of Veronica. That would change.

I went back to Laura with a more open mind about the Atlantis stuff and was now actually very excited to know more around her memories. This was my first real experience around communicating with a person who is not really human, but a multidimensional cosmic being. That is the best description I can give of Laura because she has never, since my first dealings with her, ever acted as one would expect a normal human being to act.

She may be in a human body, but she lives totally in the moment, never thinking, never in the past or future, but always allowing whatever comes to her in the moment to be her guidance.

As events unfolded I would learn that she sees energy just as easily as we see the physical world. She can see your soul and who you really are in the higher realms—the truth of your soul, as opposed to the illusion of character created here in the third dimensional world. In essence, she could see the parts of me that were in truth about myself, and the parts that weren't!

This meeting began my transformation with Laura as my guide. The unveiling of all the things I had created around the self that I thought I was: the emotional turmoil or dark places in my soul that I was afraid to visit. All would come up piece by piece, sometimes with ease, but more often kicking and screaming as I chose to see the mirror of myself reflected in her. Such is the work she is here to do, and she has helped multitudes of others besides me.

Yoga itself is a fascinating practice. The poses in yoga can unlock energetic blocks or knots within the physical body. Energy always happens first, then it moves into physicality and thus into matter. Energetic blockages are always the summoning of energy by a person, and then the person not allowing the energy to flow easily through them. Usually this happens as a result of a limiting thought or judgment that is at odds with the new thought you are trying to entertain.

For myself, I wanted to move into a higher more expanded awareness of energy and the limitless expansion of the universe. A grand concept to be sure, but at the same time, I was holding very definite ideas around how I understood the world and the way I felt it should operate. I was holding onto old patterning around what was right and wrong in pretty much every area of my life. Compound that by cellular memory from all the lives you have ever lived in human form. All that patterning from each life creates polarized thoughts on everything you have ever experienced. Beauty being better than ugliness, rich being better than poor, certain foods are bad, other foods are good. If one really pays attention to one's thoughts, one will find that they are polarized around pretty much every thought they have. This was quite a realization for me.

Laura was my first real live day-to-day experience when it came to the dismantling of me and who I thought I was. It was exhausting. It was amazing. Then it would be exhausting again. And so it went as I stubbornly allowed this woman who was my guide to steer me out of the depths of my illusions. She was alternately ruthless in her compassion and steadfast in her commitment and love as she helped me traverse the opening of ever newer levels.

I was excited with my new found guide and her amazing abilities. I was very curious as to what she could see and remember from other lives we had lived. I was sure she would want to share this information with me. Yet another lesson to be learned. She told me to mediate on such things and see what came to me.

I was to experience much of this in the future; I realized that I would have to do all the work in terms of revealing myself to myself. Laura would help guide me towards the emotions or situations I should look at, but the epiphanies would have to come from me. Such is the level of a great guide. They know they cannot do it for you. It must come from you. That is where the growth is. At the same time, Laura also engaged in a healing regime with me whereby she would enter my energy field and affect the actual physical DNA that was creating the cancer. She holds the keys to change DNA. She has the ability to remove the cell memories that were creating the disease, and as they were removed over a period of time the disease could no longer hold itself in my energy field. The result of this energetic work translated into the physical diminishing of the cancer in my body and its ability to be created again.

Laura's abilities and the work she is here to do are expanding exponentially. You can find information regarding Laura and her role here for humanity at this time by going to any of her sites. You can find her information at any of the following places:www.thequeenoflight.comwww.iamthequeenoflight.comwww.pleiadiandelegate.comwww.youtube.com/Pleiadiandelegatewww.facebook.com/PleiadianDelegate

She is profound in her ability to bring harmony to all who wish to move into the elevated frequencies of this time. She is dedicated in her desire to bring new awareness of the ever-changing energies to all with her teachings at this moment of transition for planet Earth.

Dolphins/Dolphin Energy Crystal Waters

The emergence of my awareness of dolphins and their role here on the planet—and my connection with them—came about as a result of my experiences with Laura.

Early in our relationship, a situation arose around a friend of my daughter's that required some drastic decisions on my part. I had a very revealing and intense dream about this person while I was on a cruise in the Caribbean. It was a sort of warning dream, very vivid, and I was left with a sense of great urgency. I procrastinated a bit around doing something about it because this person was not in any way aware of anything in the metaphysical world like I was experiencing. Quite the contrary. This person was very much of a logical and scientific bent.

While I was pondering what to do, an actual life threatening-situation transpired for this person, and thus I realized that I had to say something to them—which I was being asked to do so. How to go about this? I really did not understand what it was all about. I just felt the intense feeling that I had to do something. I eventually called Veronica and gave them this person's name. She told me this person was ill and needed an energy alignment as soon as possible. That they were heading towards something serious that would manifest in the physical very soon. They confirmed to me that this person's higher consciousness was contacting me because I was aware and would listen. That it was appropriate for me to speak to them.

I took it upon myself to have a meeting with this person and give them my awareness of all that I knew. I trusted that it would make some sense to them on some level and hoped that this action would absolve me of my responsibility. Oh, if only it were that easy!

The friend decided to talk to Veronica personally. She did impress upon them to have the energy alignment, as she stated it no less than twenty times during the call. This person felt it would be a dire tempting of fate to not do so. I was inspired to have them ask Veronica if Laura could do the energy alignment—I had no idea what such a thing involved, or who could do it. Veronica said yes, Laura would know what to do. So I explained the whole thing to Laura who confirmed that she understood what was needed, and she did it. Laura's ability to see the aura around a person and to manipulate energy allowed her to fix the huge hole that was encompassing this person's entire solar plexus area. She agreed that something very dire would have happened in the physical had they not seen to it—and so an unpleasant manifestation was averted.

This was the beginning of the awareness and benefit of having activations from Laura. Veronica informed me that Laura's abilities to work with physical human DNA from the energetic realms were profound. She was already doing weekly healing sessions on me, and this interaction opened a new door for more advanced activations of my soul blueprint. Laura, like all of us, is expanding and reaching new levels continuously. Unlike the rest of us, she is consciously aware of herself on all levels of existence. This was an exciting new development. This experience showed her what new levels of healing she could reach in helping people with these activations. So of course, I wanted one.

In hindsight, it was quite interesting how things came about through coincidence. This is always a sign that energy is moving into new areas of experience. A couple of days before my first activation, after yoga was finished, Laura showed us a coin and asked if any of us owned it. It was from Iceland and had two dolphins on it. None of us recognized it, and Laura said she had never seen it before and was wondering where it had come from.

My first activation was how the dolphins came through. I cannot speak of other's activations— they are personal and confidential—but I can give you a sense of them through my own experience, and you can, of course, see many testimonials on Laura's websites.

I felt pretty relaxed, and Laura talked and described to me the entire time what was transpiring from her level of perception. I felt a bit of energy buzzing through me at times, but not much more than that. Laura described what she was doing and what she was seeing: most of it was brilliant light, some white, some purple. She could see where my aura was protectively pulled in around my heart area and solar plexus. She smoothed everything out and then went into my blueprint, which makes sense to her, but at that time, not to me! Again, her websites can provide better information on her services and how they are performed.

At the end of my session, after I stood up, she looked startled.

"There are two dolphins around you," she said. Okay. By now I should be used to this sort of thing. That is how the dolphins first came through. Apparently they were very happy.

After this activation, I started to have intense blasts of a noise that I can only identify as *sonar* go through my head. I have had it happen about four or five times since that initial session. There is no mistaking it—it just about takes my head off it is so loud. A very unusual experience. Also, after this activation, I started having dreams about dolphins. One very dramatic one that had me standing in a room with a glass wall fronting an ocean; there was a pod of dolphins right in front of me in the water, and they rose up into the air, very large, and crashed into the water, which smashed the windows all around me. It was a very intense dream.

As a result of this dream, the next time I talked with Veronica, I asked about the dolphin aspect that seemed to be coming forward. She explained to me that I have lived a life as a dolphin for the purposes of studying their healing techniques. They are fifth-dimensional beings, very ancient and advanced. They are helping humanity at this very important time. She said I have come to their attention and that they were trying to break down barriers in order to be able to communicate with me through the dream, and that they are helping to heal me. She added that my unfolding life's work in the future will be connected with the dolphins.

Laura has had various encounters and visions around my work with the dolphins, and she was guided to show me how to create crystal waters—a method by which the dolphin's enhance the water through the crystals with their energies that can move through me as a result of my abilities as a healer here in physical form due to my life as a dolphin. All lives are connected. This one is just a little more unusual for the average understanding, but I feel the truth of it, and feel very happy with their connection to me.

I have since created the various crystal waters using each crystal for their specific healing ability. For example, a person wanting to calm themselves and be in harmony would want amethyst crystal water. An overarching healing crystal water would be rose quartz—it is the most powerful of all healing crystals. I have created many specific crystal waters for individual healing requirements. I look forward to the further adventures that will unfold in my life with dolphins.

Chapter 29.
FEMININE AND MASCULINE ENERGIES

Feminine energy is located in the right hemisphere of the brain and controls the left side of the physical body. Masculine energy is located in the left hemisphere of the brain and controls the right side of the body.

Feminine energy is considered to hold the aspects of intuition, instinct, knowing, unconditional love, compassion, understanding, nurturing and helpfulness. This energy is passive in nature, with a peacefulness emanating from heart centered awareness. The left side of the body represents receptivity, a taking in of feminine energy, reflective of the woman, the mother. Feminine energy is represented by the moon.

Masculine energy is considered to hold the aspects of action, logical mind, *just the facts* sort of rational thinking, structure, confidence, strength and courage. This energy is dominant or active in nature and comes primarily from mind-centered thinking. Masculine energy is represented by the sun.

Both of these polarities in energy are required to be in harmony within a person for a balance of optimum health within the body, mind and spirit. When I first understood this, it became very clear to me that everything that went wrong with my physical body always happened on the left side. Pretty much every ache, illness or injury during my life has manifested on my left side. This points to the areas of emotional trauma that are wanting to be integrated and released. I was denying my feminine aspects, or in a state of non-receiving of love and nurturing of the self. The deep sense of unworthiness that accompanied not only this life but other past lives locked in my cellular memory all resulted in the manifestation of the various physical ailments on my left side, which culminated drastically in my developing breast cancer.

The predominance of masculine energy on the planet—which has been in effect for a very long time—is coming to an end. A balancing of both polarities on the earth is what the new age of 2013 and beyond is all about. Everyone must integrate the feminine energies in order to be able to move forward with the heightened vibrations of the earth which is moving into a golden age.

A balance of divine feminine energy and divine masculine energy is the absolute universal requirement for all who wish to move into oneness with source energy, to ascend in an enlightened state or a self-realized state while still being here in a physical body.

The balancing of the two polarities of feminine and masculine energies in the physical body will bring you feelings of being healed, a wholeness, a happiness and joy that emanate an overall sense of peacefulness.

Chapter 30.
THE EGO AND EMOTIONS

The ego is the driving force and authority of physical third dimensional experience. One of the best books I have encountered that describes the ego and its hold on a person is Eckhart Tolle's *The Power of Now.*

The upcoming new earth energy is about moving out of ego *mind energy* and moving into *heart energy* which is acceptance and trust of the higher self that operates from a level of intuition coming from universal knowledge, as opposed to the ego which operates from separation and strategies around survival.

The ego operates from the thinking mind, always projecting into the past or imagining possible futures. Living from the perspective of the higher self involves living in the present moment and being content with whatever is happening in that moment. This sounds like a very clear and concise concept on the surface, and it is, but is much harder to practice in day-to-day third dimensional reality—I can tell you this from experience!

To live in the moment requires a belief and trust in something intangible beyond the body and physical matter. For most humans, who are entrenched in the modern religion of science, if something can't be measured, then it doesn't exist. My whole journey has been based on my intuition around my knowing that I am meant to live this experience and that, by doing so, something larger than myself will come out of it. That something larger is a knowing that, by sharing my experience of how I healed myself from cancer, I can and will benefit many people. I am learning from it, but it also affects others around me.

The smaller self is the person that I am in physical life. The person who allows all that happens to happen without trying to reason, struggle, or deny any of it. I am trusting that a higher force—which knows more than my waking self here in third dimensional reality—is running the show from a more expanded view of life in this universe.

It is a great show of hubris to think that we here in physical bodies can control and guide the beautiful tapestry of life in the universe from our limited perspective as humans. The marrying of intellect with intuition is the most successful recipe for living a life of flow in harmony with the cosmic plan. The higher self is the unmanifested version of you which resides in the higher realms of vibration, and it is always seeking new experiences on the material plane for the expansion of the soul.

We all plan our lives in minute detail before incarnating on this physical earth. If a person just lived in the present moment and did not judge, fear or try to control anything that happened to them in each and every day—if instead they just allowed all to be what it is in each and every moment and knew it all to be perfect for the unfolding of their soul's path—they would live in cosmic flow.

If a person never had thoughts around the health of their body and completely trusted the body to do what it organically is programmed to do, there would never be a moment of ill health. One would have a much more carefree and joyful ride through their earthly experience.

As I came to understand this, there came a point where I had to surrender to the belief that what was happening to me was by my own design. By allowing it all to unfold and observe it, I knew that I would learn from each moment of the experience revealing itself. I completely trusted my body to heal itself. Of course this undertaking is made easier when you truly believe that you are not just this body and that your consciousness is eternal and that the person you know to be *you* never really dies. I put myself to the ultimate test of this. I have been living with my mortality and my belief in immortality ever since. I trust my soul, and it has not let me down.

WHAT ABOUT PHYSIC SURGERY

I am here, three years later, having removed a potentially terminal diagnosis of cancer from my body with nothing more than my belief that you create your own reality. I held firmly to my intention and dedication to change the energy of illness and despair into one of hope and finally joy and health.

I write about my experience from a sincere desire to impart all that I have lived and learned to the courageous hearts of others wanting to discover and take back their own power. Every person on the planet has all they need inside of them to be a sovereign energy operating in love and bliss, the way humans were designed to be. Now is the time for all humans to remember who they are and live a physical life with full knowledge of their spiritual heritage.

Fear

This is probably the most important topic in the whole book. I have mentioned it many times already. Fear is what every soul on the planet needs to overcome and let go of. It is directed from the ego, and it keeps all of us firmly locked in the linear. Fear can be direct and palpable, or it can be sneaky, subtle and sly. The ego is a jealous master and will not easily be pushed aside. In the physical, we actually need the ego; it is part of our makeup here in the human condition. It stops us from doing stupid things that can end our lives prematurely. However, in order to bring in the levels of awareness from the higher realms that are wanting to come through each of us at this time and to master such elevated levels in the physical body here on earth, the ego must be tamed and become subservient to the higher self. This requires much attention to the deep-seated judgment and fears that are held in our emotional and mental bodies.

I had a very intense educational experience around fear and the body that highlighted part of my decision to try alternative methods for healing my body of cancer.

I had a sister-in-law who developed cancer in various parts of her body at the age of forty-two. She went on to battle, fight, and resist the ravaging illness that was going on in her body and psyche for three years.

She was a trooper, I will admit. She went along with all the recommendations from her doctors, and she was known in her city hospital for being the person who had taken the highest number of chemotherapy sessions of anyone they had ever admitted. She was determined, in every way, to beat this disease, and after suffering greatly for the most part—although there were moments between treatments where she reached a measure of good energy and respite—she died in the hospital fighting for each breath.

I admire my sister-in-law greatly, as she made her choices, which I respect, and I learned much from her journey. She was always easy with everyone who was around her, making them feel comfortable in her presence, she did not want anyone to feel bad for her.

By this time, I had quite a lot of awareness around how things are created in the physical, and respecting that everyone creates their reality, I always spoke my truth with her in the hopes of opening or unlocking a different perspective around fear and choice and such philosophical understandings that I had come to know for myself.

She, however, was here to walk her path, and I honor the road she set for herself, a steep climb to be sure. Understanding that there are no coincidences in life, this was part of her soul evolvement. It was a great example to me of what the physical manifestation of fear looks like in third dimensional reality. While she was stoic when around others, deep down she was afraid of the cancer and she did not want to die. Of course not, anyone can relate to this, and the fear of not knowing what comes after death is palpable for many. I honor my sister-in-law and her journey, and I thank her for showing me insights with great integrity that I could not otherwise have observed. It was a contributing factor to my own choices, and I appreciate her connection with me in this great experience called life.

Fear is a low vibration and has been used by global manipulators to keep us locked in drama and polarity and, therefore, prisoners to this third dimensional plane. Just look at our world today, and all you see is the mass marketing of fear. Fear about the safety of the planet, fears about the economy, fear about the weather and the global environmental crisis, fear around having the perfect image, fear around illness, a pandemic on the planet right now... need I go on?And then there is the entertainment industry, which the news media has become part of, they peddle drama and crisis as a steady diet, masquerading it as news. Most movies today are full of intense drama and fear-based plots to keep the adrenaline junkies of today enthralled. With such a steady diet of stress and mayhem, it is amazing that we are coping at all. Fear is not necessary; it is the ultimate illusion and needs to be let go of.

I believe that ninety-nine percent of the world's population would rather live in peace, harmony and happiness but think that it is not possible. The knowledge of our divine heritage as eternal beings has been a carefully guarded secret throughout time. That is all about to change. And it starts with knowing about fear, recognizing how much you are in fear in most moments of the day, and finding a way to move out of being in fear. The ultimate breaking of this limiting pattern will be the freedom of the entire planet.

This understanding and acknowledgement of fear was key to my success. Facing how much fear was running my life. For me it started the day my mother died. I hardly remember anything before that day; life was like a sweet cloud drifting along aimlessly, and I was enjoying each wonder as it came my way. I was a very present child, living in the moment until the day my life drastically altered with my first major fear: the fear of death. I have come full circle from that day, and it shaped my childhood and most of my adult life.

I was now again being asked to face this most tenacious fear, a fear held by pretty much every person on the planet. So why are we so afraid of death? Because we have been led to believe that there is only this life and no one knows what lies beyond this existence. Well, I was astounded and amazed at how much information is out there in the world today and in history in general around this very topic. It makes one wonder why such important information is not taught in schools and universities.

Many people in history have gone to great lengths and endured great sacrifice to keep this information alive. When a person starts seeking and goes looking with an open mind, there is much literature, symbols, art, and works in stone from the very beginnings of time to support the eternal nature of all energies within not only this universe but others as well. One only need look at the works of ancient Egyptians, Sumerians, Greeks, Incas, Mayans, Celts, and then onward in time to the Gnostics, Cathars, Templars, Free Masons, and the list goes on.

There is a fantastic book by the author Michael Newton called *Journey of Souls*. This man has a PhD and is an incredible resource on what is termed case studies of life between lives. He is a psychologist who has founded the Newton Institute, and he pioneers techniques for using hypnotherapy to take people to this state of awareness that is within each one of us. His message: No one dies. They just move into a different state of awareness. The human body is energy. Physics has determined this. Einstein's quote "Energy cannot be created or destroyed, it can only be changed from one form to another…" supports this. This is shown quite consistently with the literally thousands of people who have been a part of Michael Newton's research, and it is documented comprehensively in the various publications he has brought forward since his groundbreaking discovery early in his career. I often recommend this book to people who have lost a loved one. They always tell me it was a great help to them and helped shift their view of death greatly. It is a humorous and enlightening read. You can visit his site at www.newtoninstitute.org.

Fear is a low vibration and therefore keeps you locked in limitation. Love and joy are the highest of vibrations and can unlock the secrets of the universe. We have been systematically kept in the vibration of fear so that we cannot easily access the higher vibrations that will release us from this bondage. Just look around you. There is a distinct feel of change in the world. People are starting to question why the world is in the state it is in. Time feels different. Everything is shifting. And it starts with each person realizing that they are in fear and then desiring to want to change this. To let go of it—to trust that we can have a world of our own choosing and that it can be one that emits a vibration of harmony and by extension a life of peace and joy. This will happen as we let go of fear.

I had read about this concept and felt it to be true. I was therefore given the ultimate test of my soul in having to walk the walk around fear. I had to face my fears one by one, and move into them and transmute them, so that they could dissolve. I had to do this over and over again for a long time because I was holding tremendous fears around so many things—I am still doing it today. I have let go of many fears already, and so the task is getting easier. I am getting happier, lighter and healthier with each and every moment of fear that I recognize in myself and subsequently let go of.

How do you recognize when you are in fear? Sometimes it is obvious, and sometimes it is not obvious at all—sometimes it is downright buried. The obvious fears, such as the fear of death, fear of suffering, fear of being inadequate, those are easy to see in oneself. But how do you let them go? Well, you have to move into them and acknowledge that you are holding the fear in the first place. Admitting this is hard for some people. We all hold ideas of who we think we are.

We spend a lifetime creating the person we think we are, or think we *should be*, and as time moves on, we are totally encased in the illusion of the self we have created. This is the ego at its finest. Who wants to admit that they are afraid of dying, or suffering in any way. Who wants to admit that they are not really that great at their job, or that they really don't enjoy the work they are doing? It's easier to forget about such things and distract ourselves with other ways of creating more of the person we think we should be.

We distract ourselves in so many ways. We spend our time watching television and online living a virtual reality rather than engaging in real-life experience, such as being out in nature. Drinking alcohol, taking drugs, eating to excess. Everyone wants a life of comfort that is uncomplicated. Easy. How did we get to be so diminished? Where is the passion and zest for life and adventure? Most cannot remember when they felt alive and full of enthusiasm for life. We are living in a risk adverse world. Risk is where all the fun, excitement and growth is.

When I was faced with my physical life being on the line, I had to make some really honest observations about who I was and how I had gotten to this point. Where was my passion for existence—I felt a great heaviness around everyday life. I had to determine how I was going tackle this terminal diagnosis and how would it define me. Because I was in fear in the beginning, I will not kid you. I was more afraid of suffering, if truth be told. I understood that I was an immortal energy, but it is easy to have such beliefs when they are shrouded in the ever expansive nature of time and philosophy. My time had come. I was being asked to live my philosophy. So I had to ante up and say to myself:*Do I really believe that I am an immortal being whose consciousness cannot die, and whose body is just a vessel that encompasses the spirit which at some point moves on to another form of existence?*The answer was yes.

Then I had to ask myself:*Do I trust that I am divinely guided in all moments and do I trust that the universe always brings me my highest experience if I let go and surrender. Can I allow this even if it means I must suffer?*Again, I received a yes. I knew in my heart that I was meant to heal myself. This was my intuition and my truth. So, from that point onwards, I allowed myself to trust that all would be as it was meant to be, and that meant I would not know what was going to happen, but I trusted that it would be the best outcome for me.

This released me from having to take mental action, from having to feel I had to be in control of any part of this. I knew from that moment on that I would be guided in each moment as to what I should do about this illness. This allowed me to let go of the fear and surrender to the moment. I did not have to worry about this; there was nothing I had to think about. It would all unfold perfectly. And it has.

I have learned much in this surrendering of the fear. I now have an experiential awareness around this concept. It is not just a trust any longer, it is a certainty. A knowing. And so began the biggest and best journey of my life in this incarnation. This illness has brought to me the most miraculous and fantastic experiences that have transcended anything I have experienced in the material world thus far.

In the early days I was mainly dealing with the big fears. As time went on, though, I found that there are a multitude of little fears that are always cropping up. Some of them may seem insignificant, but on the journey to being a master of spirit in a body, many little tests arise. The format for moving out of large or small fears is really the same. The smaller fears can be a bit more elusive however.

It takes focus to be aware of when you are experiencing a small fear that wants to be recognized consciously. My initial awareness of this was I would notice I did not feel good around a specific action or encounter. This was my first indication that a fear was lurking just under the surface of my waking consciousness. It could simply be a statement someone would utter, or an action that put me off. I would have a *not good* feeling around it.

In the past, I would have just let it go, not even registering it—it would be gone that quickly. To get a sense of what I am trying to explain, pretend for a moment you have run into an old acquaintance from school. You are asked questions like: What are you doing now, where do you work? As the answers flow back and forth, the ego is usually stimulated—inevitably, one party or the other feels like they are not measuring up. Your friend may have become highly successful and has informed you that their progeny have become doctors and lawyers. In contrast, your children may be working at the local grocery store. Or vice versa—you may be the one with the doctors and lawyers. This is an interesting experience from both sides and each person has a lesson to be learned.

It takes deep introspection around why you had a bad feeling around a chance encounter that yields to you the gold. It takes perseverance and total commitment to get to the truth around what made you feel bad and what you are fearing. Most will shy away from being so brutally honest with themselves.

First, why do you feel that somehow you are less than your friend because their children are professionals? What is really going on at the deeper levels? Well, perhaps this old school chum was great at sports and you weren't. Maybe he or she was a great student and always got a better mark on their science projects than you did. A feeling comes up on either side of not being as good, a feeling of unworthiness. Take that a little further and you are heading into a feeling of not loving yourself. There is a deeply rooted feeling of you not being lovable, and it was just stimulated by this person from your past, and your soul wants you to deal with it.

Your soul wants you to recognize that you hold this fear so that you can let it go and transmute it into a feeling of love for yourself. You do not need to judge yourself. But on some level, you just did. Most people just register for a moment that they don't feel so good around this interaction, say goodbye, and move on with their day. But something was activated deep in your psyche that wants to be released, and therefore the *feeling* should have been your barometer that something is buried and wants to come up and be recognized and let go of. This is a fear. A subtle fear but a fear nonetheless. This is the start of releasing fear, the recognition that you have one. It is a great step forward when you start recognizing that you have all these little fears that bring out judgments of the self or others that compound into a large cauldron of simmering brew waiting under the surface to keep you in misery and suffering.

As for the other side of this interaction, we are mirrors for each other; it is always a projection you are creating that mirrors your own state of fear back to you. The person who was really great at sports and good at science, is measuring their self worth by all of their achievements. They feel this defines them in a way that proves their worthiness.

Their ego is happy to list all of the accolades around their perceived successful children in a desire to further enhance their own sense of worth. If they looked into this more deeply it would reveal a false sense of who they are. They are deeply into the illusion that material goods and social status will make them feel loved. Would they be as deeply satisfied if their children were workers in the local manufacturing plant? Can they be happy just letting everything be as it is? This is the level of frequency you are trying to reveal to yourself.

It is a simple formula. Can you trust that everything and everyone is exactly where they need to be to learn the lessons their soul is here to learn—without judgment. The mundane and the divine are equal teachers. Both misery and joy are both desired experiences by the soul. There is choice in each and every moment, and usually, if you just feel what you think to be the right action for you in each moment, the outcomes will be of the highest experience for your path in the third dimension.

Resistance

On the surface, resistance can seem very much like fear, and they are certainly related. I have found, however, that resistance is usually a precursor to an underlying fear, and comes up to show you that there is something within you that needs looking at. It will usually present itself as a feeling of uncomfortableness. This could be physical or emotional.

Physically, it can come up as direct pain or an illness such as flu or perhaps a general overall feeling of fatigue. Emotionally, it can present as depression, or feelings of loneliness. A heaviness that does not allow you to be happy. It is a constriction of your emotions, or your body. Acceptance is expansion; resistance is constriction.

As you come to desire to understand the subtleties of what is happening to you on all these levels of unfolding awareness, you will find that it takes great focus and intent to want to delve into the areas of resistance and reach a point of acceptance, where you can allow your feelings and physical experiences that cause much distress in the moment. Ultimately this will be your release into peace and health on all levels.

I had my first tangible experience with resistance at the Casa in Brazil while sitting in the current. The feeling of pain that I felt in my chest and back area was my first example of how I needed to move into non-resistance. That was a very intense example. It was only in the experiencing of such a deep *now moment* that I could discern the relationship between resistance and surrender. I just allowed the pain to be; no thoughts, just observation and a letting go on a deep level. And as a result, it just went away—it was transmuted. Deep cellular memory evaporated in that moment. But then more came up, and I had to do it all over again. However, in committing to this process, the pain eventually diminished until, one day, it was gone.

Everyone on the planet is in the process of understanding that they are in resistance to pretty much everything. We will all come to master the art of allowing in our own way and time. So I can only tell it as I experience it. I have come to be quite comfortable with the ongoing situations of discomfort that come up. As I stated earlier, I find that resistance usually points to an underlying fear. The feeling comes up, you admit to yourself that there is something there, and then you go into it and see what fear comes up.

This sounds simple on the surface, but can be a bit tricky. You have to really desire to look truthfully at your own heart and be honest with yourself around what is bothering you. You have to do this over and over again. It's okay to just let the feelings come up and be with them. You don't always have to figure things out, just accept that they are there and be okay with that. Don't judge yourself. Allow yourself to feel whatever emotion wants to come up. Just let it come up. It *will* hurt. It *will* feel bad, and you *will* perhaps feel fear or heartache or shame or anger. Anything can come up from the simplest of situations over the course of a day. Just notice when you feel *not good*. Notice the resistance you hold onto in order to deal with the bad feelings. Notice the pain somewhere in your body. Notice it all, and just allow it, *feel* it, and love yourself in spite of whatever it brings up for you.

This will allow it to be transmuted, and you will get lighter and lighter, more peaceful. Eventually more experiences of joy and bliss will grace your heart. And you will *know*, in these moments, the amazing work you have done has yielded results. You will know that you are on to something that works. This is a very courageous act. And as you get more comfortable with this process, you will come to have complete confidence in your ability to handle anything that comes into your realm of experience because, whether it is a good feeling or a not so good feeling, you will also come to know that you create them all and that you can then choose what you want to experience in a more focused way in each moment.

It starts with recognizing that you are in resistance on many levels and that you now intend to move into a state of acceptance of what you have created. Eventually, through the art of allowing, all desired experiences will come your way. You create your reality. All of it. And an understanding that you enjoy contrasting experiences allows you to have a sense of acceptance that, on a higher level, your soul is learning, and that the perceived unhappy experiences are no less desired that the happy ones.

Surrender

The subtleties of surrender. This is a simple idea with a large field of variables that keep coming up to confuse and trap you in your ego. Simply put, surrendering is letting go and trusting that all is well in all of creation, in each and every moment. This statement applies regardless of what is happening to you at any given time. Now, when you are told you just won $50,000 in the lottery, surrendering to the moment is pretty easy. Hearing that a parent has suddenly died, worrying about a child, or being told you have a terminal illness, well now these are not so easy. We tend to judge situations as being good or bad. Being in judgment keeps us from surrendering to the moment. Truly letting go of judgment and allowing whatever wants to be—well this takes some deep emotional awareness. A trust that there is order in the chaos.

We have been taught to try to control and handle any situation that may arise in our lives from the perspective of the mind. So each and every moment that is unfolding in our lives ultimately becomes judged by the mind as either a good experience or a bad experience. A desirable experience versus a not so desirable experience. No one would argue that feeling good is better than feeling bad. But how could we ever know what felt good if we hadn't felt something that didn't feel good. This is the basis of polarity and the name of the game in our universe. As long as you are in polarity you are not in surrender. Because surrendering means that you trust that you have a larger plan that is unfolding in perfect harmony with the true desires of your soul. There is really no way you can get it wrong, and therefore all experiences are in divine order. When you get out of your own way and stop trying to control what is occurring in your life and accept everything as being perfectly orchestrated from the higher part of yourself—ultimately from source energy—you are in surrender.

For me, this meant accepting my breast cancer as being in perfect harmony with my soul's desire to have this experience. Now it took many twists and turns along the way in my adhering to and understanding this concept. In the beginning, it was pretty scary. Okay, let go and let it all be what it wants to be. What did that mean? Was I going to have to suffer? How would I handle that? Was I going to die? How would that actually unfold, and how peaceful could I be around that in each and every day and hour, not knowing how things were going to unfold.

Early on, I wrestled with my understanding of what surrender really felt like, and I waffled back and forth in my commitment to stay surrendered. I would suddenly notice myself having expectations around some of my healing modalities. When things would be going really well, I would feel very empowered and would feel that soon I would be healed and everyone would see how successful I had been—and this became a goal. Then I would have small setbacks, and I would have to readjust my thinking around what I was doing, and then I would suddenly realize that I had fallen back into coming from my mind and trying to control the situation. So back to surrender! Truly surrendering. This would mean going deep into my heart and soul and trusting and letting go to whatever wanted to happen—the worst case scenario or the best case scenario—not caring about any outcomes, just knowing that whatever was unfolding was perfect.

This requires you to not care what anyone thinks of you, regardless of what action or non-action you choose in any moment. As soon as I entered wholly into this, I could feel my body ease. I felt more peaceful and then any subtle pain would subside. Then I would start the whole cycle again. I would be in surrender and feel great and then slowly, incrementally, as each day's life experiences distracted me from observing myself in each moment, I would again find myself having desires and expectations around how the journey should be.

The ego is a tenacious master and will constantly wrestle with you for control. However, I have finally noticed that, when I feel great, I am in surrender mode, and therefore it became much easier to recognize when I wasn't because I would feel stressed or start to have discomfort or subtle pain in my body. Again, back to surrender.

And so the pendulum swung, and I slowly became more balanced and peaceful with my understanding and acceptance of my path. Today, as I write this, I have no fear of death. I am truly blessed with this experience. It has given me a feeling of sincere gratitude in letting go of any fears I have concerning my own mortality. I am now excited to see what eventually comes of this creative adventure of mine. It matters not whether I will stay on the planet and continue to evolve and experience each moment from a perspective of allowing or decide to leave and move on to other things in the universe. I am in constant enjoyment of each and every moment, knowing that I have perfectly created each of them.

A friend of mine told me a story that I could really relate to. It was about a woman who lived on the west coast of Canada. She was well known as a person who lived a very holistic lifestyle, used alternative medicine, and was very committed to a natural healing approach to life. Two of her daughters became naturopathic doctors. All of a sudden, she was diagnosed with breast cancer. She was determined to heal herself, and over a period of twelve months, she had travelled to many places in the world trying to access healing practices that she felt would take this from her. In the end, after great expense, none of them worked and she barely made it back to Canada where she then died.

After telling me this story, my friend commented that she felt this woman had actually run from her family and friends because she felt, in some way, that she had failed in her approach to life and that being healed by alternative medicine became an obsessive goal which she felt she needed to prove to all those around her.

This story resonated with me because I could very much relate to this woman and have fallen victim to this thought process myself on more than one occasion during my journey. This goes to the depths of surrendering. I too was always a person who practiced natural healing methods and intuitively felt that this was the correct way for the planet to be heading. I knew that friends and family wondered how someone like myself ended up having cancer—I had always taken care of myself, ate healthy food, exercised, told people how to heal themselves with many natural methods. *So why did I get sick?*It scared people to think that it could get someone like myself who practiced all the *right* things to prevent illness. I could easily have fallen into this mindset myself. It did lurk in the back of my mind, I will admit. However, I had a strong belief in my soul's ability to guide me through this, and so I trusted that, while I did not know at this point why all these things were happening to me, they were happening for a very good reason and that someday I would know why I had chosen this experience.

I accepted that it didn't matter if, in the physical world, people had thoughts that I would fail. It didn't matter to me that my beliefs would be questioned by many of them—it was not my business what other people thought of me. I had to let go of the fear that the ego was creating around the person that I felt I had been to this point—the personality that I had created thus far—and let go of who I thought I should be. Letting go of the old pattern of who you are is like a small death, and the person you become through that experience is like a birth. The birth of a new person. The real essence of who you really are. Who you came here to be.

I knew that I was serving a greater purpose and that, someday in the future, it would be realized on the planet—people would come to know that they have the power to heal themselves. But we have to get from here to there, and patience is required as we pioneer our way forward.

I realized that I must accept that it may not happen in the timeline I perceive it should—realized that I had to let go of any attachments I was holding around my part in all of this. Allowing and surrendering are subtle arts that take some mastering. But when you truly get there, you will feel at peace and will be in perfect harmony with your soul. A very great lesson. I am thankful for the continuing experience of surrender. It is ongoing.

Acceptance

Acceptance is a total surrender to what is. In any moment. Whatever is going on is meant to be going on. No judgment around it as to whether it is good or bad, right or wrong. Whatever is IS.

This is very hard for most of us to practice here at this time on planet Earth—we have been living in a world of polarity, a world that has been measured in black and white for eons. Just think for a moment of all the ideas you hold that place you on one side or the other of any experience. That murder is wrong, or that helping the poor is right. You may feel war is horrendous. Or that gay marriage is okay, or not okay. These are blatant examples. As a species we are pretty much polarized on everything.

The earth is changing, and we are being asked to perceive what is happening from a very different perspective. The world is being confronted with a new understanding that is asking each person to become aware of—and to trust—that all that is happening in the universe is in perfect order and that there is a beautiful plan that is unfolded from the higher levels of awareness, a plan that we, in our multidimensionality, are also a part of.

Here in the physical body, at this moment, most of us do not have the level of awareness that transcends this place and time because the larger picture transcends time and space. That is all about to change.

Now is the time we are starting to remember and to become aware that we have planned this all along. Therefore, we are at a culmination point of a process that has been a long time in the making by us.

Acceptance is the final step in the letting go of us thinking of ourselves as separate from all things. It is a realization that we are just energy, enjoying the experience as spirit in form, and that we are evolving into a being that will have the full knowledge and awareness of the vastness of all that we are while still in the physical body.

This is what the time of 2013 and beyond is all about: a revolution in consciousness, a marriage of the form and formless parts of ourselves. The embodiment of the vastness of our spirit in the physical body. It starts with acceptance of the process, your awareness that, as a being in physical form, you are perfect and that you do not have to do anything other than let it unfold.

This is the quickest route to getting there. The realizing that there is nowhere you have to get to—that you are already there. When you are in acceptance, then you are okay with whatever is going on. No fears, no judgment, no ideas of right or wrong. All experience is desired. Period. That will set you free. That's quite a leap for most of us, but we are well on our way, and things are unfolding perfectly. I feel this whenever I am in acceptance. It just feels right. No letting the mind get in the way. No letting the ego make you fear or wonder what is it all about? Just a letting go, and trusting that you have this all from the higher level of your soul. Your soul will never let you down. And acceptance of its ability to guide you is a very wonderful feeling.

Chapter 31.
LOVE AND ASCENSION

There are only two vibrations: love and fear. You can usually tell which one you are vibrating to if you feel within yourself at any moment. Fear feels awful. Love feels wonderful. It is really that simple though the mind can keep you in a state of distraction or confusion with all the varying degrees of feeling between these two states.

Fear can be present in your awareness as despair, anger, shame, or pain; and love can be present as hope, joy, bliss and ultimately ecstasy.

Be aware of which vibration are you consciously choosing in each moment. Check within your body and heart constantly to see what you are vibrating to. Love or fear. You will always know, and it is a great practice to keep yourself in the present moment, by checking in often and reminding yourself that it is all choice. You can choose, in any moment, to recognize whether you are having fearful negative thoughts, or positive loving thoughts.

If you check in and realize that you are vibrating with negativity, whether it is obvious or subtle, then realize in that moment that you have the ability to change the pattern of your thoughts into positive thoughts that allow more love to flow through you.

This can be done by recognizing that you are feeling a certain way and allowing the feelings to come up, honoring them without judging yourself, feel them deeply and let them go. Never keep fearful uncomfortable thoughts at bay; deal with them, and let them move through you. I have come to a point where I love to feel good because I remember how it felt to feel awful. I always notice now when I move out of flow and peacefulness. I just don't feel good. And the price of losing that beautiful feeling is too high a price for me to pay these days. I always recognize when I am out of harmony and move back into that state by facing what is causing me to feel off, and surrendering to the moment—allowing what wants to come forward with total acceptance.

There is an inspirational movie that illustrates many of the concepts involved in loving yourself and how this acceptance of yourself unconditionally can heal a person. It is called "You Can Heal Your Life", and it was created by Louise Hay. This woman has been a pioneer from the first time she came across the concept of creating one's own reality. I heard her speak about this at a conference and how the concept had profoundly influenced her. She has been a maverick in bringing forward this philosophy in her efforts to help people realize their own ability to affect their life through their belief that they create their own circumstances and experiences through their vibration and alignment with positive energy. She has written books and created her own publishing company (Hay House) which publishes many books in the metaphysical and spiritual/self-help field. You can watch this very visually enlightening movie by going to the official site at www.youcanhealyourlifemovie.com.

The moment of what is termed *ascension* is now upon us all. It is important to understand that you have created all of this experience from the higher levels of yourself that transcend this life. Look at this life as your own movie, created by you, starring you. If you change the way you feel inside of you, the outside world will change to reflect your new vibration. It is the way the universe works. I have put this to the test and found that it works. Put it to the test yourself, don't just take my word for it. It was one of the practices that allowed me to heal myself. The holographic field that we see as our everyday world is in a constant change of fluctuating timelines that reflect the inner world of each being on the planet. This is called multidimensionality, and while it is very hard for one to comprehend this concept with the linear mind at this point, all of us will move into the intuitive knowing and remembering of this way of being that is our natural destiny. Change what goes on inside of you, and the outside will change. One of the most effective ways to bring yourself into flow and into a state of harmony is to feel gratitude or appreciation in your heart. Just think of something that you felt grateful for; move that feeling into your heart and hold it. You will notice that you can feel the difference in your vibration, and your outside world will change to reflect this. We are all experiencing our own personal awakening at this time. The experiential meeting of all that we are in the cosmos, coming together in full awareness, in the vibration of love, in the physical body: this is ascension. All is in perfect order. Enjoy the ride, and don't be afraid.

Being in the Body

It is important for a person to be firmly grounded in their body. The body is an earthy physical vehicle. It is the denseness of matter vibrating at the third dimensional level. The upcoming shift on planet earth—the consciousness revolution that will bring about ascension—is all about bringing your soul awareness into the physical body. Spirit into form.

This is quite an undertaking—it has never been done before—and we have all been working towards this for quite some time from an eternal perspective. All the lives you have ever lived are coming into a completion stage at this moment in time and space. Even time will flow differently from now on. Many people have noticed this. I hear it all the time, even from those who have not awakened yet. They notice that time has somehow changed from the way they used to experience it.

This is a gradual undertaking being orchestrated from the higher realms in cooperation with every person on the planet. Everyone is doing this at their own pace in the perfect unfolding with their own soul plan. No one has gotten it wrong.

Some will wake up earlier in order to help others by sharing with them what they have already experienced. This will help ease the masses into the transformation that is on track for the whole planet. You see this happening already.

One of the most important things to realize is that, to experience this new golden age, you must be in the body. Happily, trustingly, and joyfully in your body. So it is high time that everyone start being as good to their body as they can. Otherwise, you are going to experience the shift as a rough ride!

I set my own soul plan up so that I would have no other choice but to pay attention to this time, and particularly my body. I was not at all grounded in my body when I was diagnosed with cancer. Obviously! I was very open in my higher chakra's, but closed in my lower ones, which are the chakra's most associated with your connection to the earth. I did not trust my body at that time—I actually feared it, worrying that it was going to let me down. I was not in a state of loving my body.

Now on the other side of this experience, I appreciate and love my body unconditionally. I know it is in co-creation with me as I move into this time of change, and I trust it implicitly to be the perfect vehicle for my spirit. We are a team, and I know it knows how to be in perfect health. This is the intention I hold, and my body responds to that intention, just as it is designed to do. It is really that simple. It is fear that gets in the way of the body being able to naturally do its job. If you let go of trying to affect your body from the mind and the worries it holds around the condition of your body, it will always be in a state of health. It can be no other way. Just let go. Thank your body and feel sincere appreciation for it whenever you can. That vibration you are sending it is all it needs to know. All will be well.

Chapter 32.
GUIDANCE

You have heard me mention several times how I have been guided along this path by energies from the spiritual realms. Anything that is not in a body, or form, is in the spirit realms, or formless. As a polarity universe, everything has to have an opposite. So we have form and formless co-existing side by side. One is visible to us, the other is not.

Guidance comes from the formless side of the fence. From the deepest part of the soul. Often this guidance is coming from higher versions of ourselves—versions residing in the spiritual realms and with access to universal information.

They can see what you have planned for yourself as the highest life plan you can experience, and they are trying to help you to stay on track. You are an aspect or fragment in human form of a much larger energy that is still you. When you come into physical form, there is a forgetting of all that you planned for this life. Every one of us has guides to help us stay the course of achieving our highest destiny, yet we often go astray when the going gets tough.

Our desire—from the initial life plan we created on the other side— was to have a deep experience on some life theme that we are always working on. Getting off the life plan happens quite a lot due to free will. Then we start to feel like our lives have gone horribly wrong, and we can become despondent or disillusioned and often this is when disease or disaster can strike. This is also when we have the greatest opportunity for soul growth. It is a matter of who are you going to be in this situation of adversity you have created. You have only to ask for help and guidance. Asking for guidance from our own personal guides will always be pure and in our best interest. Asking for help from individuals who channel energies from the other side, or who practice energy medicine while being human themselves... well, that can be a bit trickier.

It's important to understand the level of awareness of various beings from the non-corporeal realms. Just because they are not in a body does not mean they are all-wise and all-knowing. Just like on earth, in the spirit realms there is wise guidance and not-so-wise guidance. It is very important to run everything you experience and all advice that appears to come your way as opportunities through your own filter of what *feels* right to you. Remember that the most important lesson everyone on the earth is learning, at this point and time, is that to contribute to the evolution of humanity is to be sovereign unto yourselves.

You do not really need to ask anyone outside of yourself for answers. All answers reside within you, if you can only trust and access this awareness. That means asking your own soul for clarity about whether something is for you or isn't. I did this each and every time I made a choice about my healing. From something as simple as deciding on a supplement, to which doctor felt right, to whether or not I should travel to Brazil, etc. Because the overarching test you will want to employ with any healing modality or experience that looks like it is being offered to you is this: *does it feel right?* Do you feel good about it? Because anything that feels good to you, makes you feel happy or excited means you are going in the right direction. Anything that causes you to feel *off* in some way, or that doesn't settle well with you, or makes you feel bad, is telling you that it is not in your highest interest. I employed this test even with my many conversations with the entity Veronica, and also all others who helped heal me energetically. Most of the guidance that I acted upon came to me in ways that felt perfect. I just *knew* it was something I had to do. That should be the litmus test by which you act.

If you are not sure, ask for guidance to be clearer. Ask them to send you a stronger sign that you will recognize. It is helpful to clarify that you want only energies of the highest intention for *your* highest experience to help you at this time. Something to that effect, which sends a clear intention from you. Then lower vibrational energies will not engage with you. You create your reality, and that means you get to decide if you want guidance along your path.

Your guides will respect your desire to choose any experience, and that means so-called perceived *bad* experiences. You see, from the spiritual perspective, you are eternal, and you never really die, and you are here in a body for the purpose of experiencing contrast, and so you get to decide how intense that experience may have to be. When you consciously realize this is how your reality works—that you are not a victim to random circumstance—you will want to focus and fine tune your experiences to ones that will be more pleasant. You will know which couriers of divine guidance are of the highest vibration because their message will usually be one of self-empowerment! You always have to ask for guidance and then get out of the way because they love it when you ask them for help!

Dreams

Everyone dreams. Whether you remember them or not. The dreamworld is a place where your spirit goes and does other things that you usually have no awareness of in your everyday waking consciousness of physical reality. Yet sometimes you can catch glimpses of these other realities when you wake up and remember your dreams. This involves the multidimensional realms.

Most people think that dreams come from the mind, and while the mind can play a part, that is a simplistic explanation. You often will resolve issues that occurred during your day in your sleep at night. These situations are obvious; there is a relationship to what you did during your day and a direct reflection of it from the dream.

The larger overarching significance of the dreamworld that most people are not aware of is its ability to show you multidimensional aspects of yourself. You are experiencing yourself in a multitude of times and places simultaneously within your experience as a soul. The soul operates on many higher levels, and you are a part of your soul, focused here in third dimensional reality for the purposes of being you. The you that you know is only part of the whole soul that is also you. And you are in many places inhabiting many forms. A bit confusing for sure. This is how the universe operates, and all incarnated on planet earth have chosen to come here to be in separation and forget the larger part of who they are so as to be able to have an authentic experience to expand the soul. If you remembered who you were in the larger scope of your consciousness, then it would not be a *real* experience. Like knowing the end of the movie before watching it. Or reading the last page of a book first.

Yours dreams can give you valuable insights and information if you start to pay attention to them. I have a great system going on in the dream world. I am aware of myself in other places and times. Often I am the person I am in this life, with most of the same characters, yet in a different place in the world, or a different city. For example, I often dream of a city that is the same city I currently live in, yet it has a totally different infrastructure and layout. I have dreamed of this place many times, and in this alternate place, I am familiar with where things are in the city, and which restaurants and stores I prefer. Upon waking, I realize that it is a totally different place than the one I experience here in my conscious life. Sometimes I am aware of both places simultaneously within the dream, I will think as I am walking down a street: *This is not like the place I live in.* I also have a reality where I am a male around the age of twenty in an Arab country. I have dreamed of this more than once, and it felt like who I am here, only I looked at myself in a mirror once in the dream and saw a young man staring back at me. It was quite interesting, I can tell you. I was aware of who I am here, and what I look like, but there it was in the mirror—another person's face. These would be considered concurrent or parallel lives.

I also dream of other worlds. I have seen various alien featured people in my dreams. They seem familiar to me in some way. Often I will know who the alien is from this life. It could be a family member, but they look totally different in the dream. Sometimes you have composite features show up in people you know. For example, your Caucasian sister may look like she usually does but have oriental shaped eyes. This is your cosmic awareness that has information of all lives you have ever lived and all universal knowledge showing you part of another reality this person is also a part of. I almost always know who the person in my dream is in this life, even when they are of a different race or gender. I can sense who they are, even when they look totally different.

I have many dreams that are prophetic—that is to say I dream about it and then it happens. I have had dreams where I have been shown crystals and dreams where I have been shown how multidimensionality actually works. That was quite a mind-blowing experience that cannot be described with words. Often in dreams, you will get information that comes as a block of knowing. I call these downloads. You observe something and have an instant knowing of a wealth of information around it that just comes to you all at once. I encourage all to have an open-minded approach to their dreams. Look at them as much more than silly stuff that goes on while you are sleeping.

I include this information on dreams even though it is personal in nature so as to encourage people to change their perspective around what they think dreams are. You can expand greatly and even help yourself heal from dreams. I have had many dreams that have shown me various states of my healing progression and have pointed out areas that I need to look at. I have shown myself supplements that I should take by dreaming about them. I have seen my body in various states of healing from the dream world. I love my dreams, and I trust what I get in them. It is important to note, however, that all physical manifestations are considered symbols, so it is helpful to know *your own symbols* and what they mean to you. For example, dreaming of an apartment or house could mean security to one person and mean a way of moving on to another. It takes a bit of trust in your intuition—your gut feeling around what message you are sending yourself from dreams. The more you observe them, the easier and more enlightening it will get.

One more interesting note is that, when you dream of yourself in another reality, to that you, YOU are the dream. Essentially everything is the dream world; the degree of difference is the ability to be awake within the dream.

Chapter 33.
VISUALIZATION

A great exercise—one that can bring quite a lot of peace and harmony to you and your physical body—is the art of visualization. The physical body and the events we experience are really just a combination of all the thoughts and emotions that we are putting out there. These thoughts are energy that ultimately manifest as solid matter and events. This is what is reflected back to us as the third dimensional world.

Our imagination is the greatest tool we have for manifesting. What you think about is what you will realize in the physical world. For example, if you worry and stress about money, having thoughts that you will never have enough, that is what you will experience in your every-day life.

If you never worry about money, feel secure, if you know that you are taken care of and that you will always have everything you need, then that is what you will experience. My sister is great at this. She never wants for anything. She is always saying how lucky she is, that she needs nothing, and she sincerely means this. She is the most giving of people, and as a result she always has money, is always winning things, etc.

Imagination and visualization are a great way to affect your emotions and ultimately the vibration you send out into the universe. So what would make you happy? What would make you feel good? Begin by daydreaming about things that make you feel wonderful. Create the feeling. This can be as simple as feeling yourself in a state of happiness and joy. What would make you feel those feelings? Imagine that.

It is the feeling that you carry within yourself that attracts the like vibration to you. This should not be stressful or limited in any way. That will constrict the energy and it will not work. Since there are no limitations in the universe, you can literally create anything you want. The only limitation is in your belief systems and the restrictions that you place upon yourself. Try this as an experiment. Think about what would make you truly happy, feel the emotions around this visualization. Then let it go. Don't let the mind come up with any limiting thoughts about how it could or would have to come about. Pretend. There are no rules or limitations in this exercise. Have trust that it will come, when it is the perfect time. You must do this from the heart with feelings of no restriction and play at it.

You will find that this yields some interesting experiences. I once cut some pictures out of various magazines that appealed to me. Years later, I noticed that most of them had come true. A couple were very specific. I remember looking at a picture of a room on a cruise ship, and realized that we had taken a cruise on that very ship had been in that very room in the picture. I had cut those pictures out five years before, put them in a file folder, and had not looked at them until about six months after our first cruise. I had read about this practice and was quite amazed to discover that it actually worked. It's great to read about these wonderful experiences, but nothing validates it like your own personal experience.

Fun

Life should be fun. Really. I think most people would agree with this statement. Yet there are a lot of people on the planet not having fun. Why is this? I believe it is because we have been brought up to be way too serious, too responsible, too accepting of the limitations that have been place upon us. It is time to free ourselves up a bit. Yes, we still have to operate in a responsible manner for many things, but it should be a major priority to choose fun in all things that we participate in.

My husband used to tell my children that *Mom was never a child.* This is a true statement, and it used to make me feel bad when he said it. Because I really was a controlling mother and a stressed out and worried parent for most of my girls' childhood. Having cancer really made me into a new person. I had to recognize parts of myself that I did not like and decide that things had to change. Then I had to actually change the way I looked at everything. Change the way you feel inside of you, and the outer world circumstances will change to reflect that feeling back to you. So today, I am much more open, and have discovered and am continuing to discover my *inner child*.

You may have noticed that children like to have FUN! So why do we lose this as we get older? Because somewhere, sometime, we were told that we had to change as we got older. This is not true. Following your bliss and making fun a priority should always be at the forefront of your life. Everyone gets to define what fun is for them. This is right up there with getting older. If you never had the concept in your mind that you age, you literally would not age. There have been some very interesting studies done around this. One that comes to mind is around a group of people who were in their late sixties, and early seventies. They were all initially checked out by doctors and had their overall health situation recorded for a comparison that would be done at the end of the study. They were taken to a town that was set up as a model of a community from the 1950s. They were asked to live for two months as if they were actually living again in that time.

They ate the foods, enjoyed the environment and culture from that time period. They were asked to pretend, act and believe as much as possible that they were anywhere between twenty and thirty years of age. They were to get into the roleplaying in their minds and in everyday practice that they were for all intents and purposes younger people living in the 1950s.

At the end of the two months they were again checked over by the same doctors, and the results were nothing less than astounding. Blood pressures that were highly elevated before were down to normal. Those who had arthritis and could hardly move were downright mobile. Some of the more elderly now had the hearts of fifty-year-olds, etc. They physically looked younger. What this study showed was the perception of being younger actually resulted in their creating a younger physical manifestation of themselves. They were in the zone. They loved the experience. They forgot that they were supposed to be old. They were having fun! Let's all consciously decide to make life more fun. It's a great choice.

Chapter 34.
FEAR OF FOOD

There is much to be said on this topic. People have increasingly become polarized around the issue of food and what is good to eat and what is not good. I commend those people who want to take charge of their health through diet and are disciplined enough to do so. It is a large subject, with many different approaches and issues.

The world abounds with books on dieting; books on different styles of cooking, cultural modes of eating, ethnic practices—and each of these have some slant on the natural ways of healing through food. People who have had success with one form of diet or healing regime around the addition or avoidance of various foods, often feel that they have *the solution.* That everyone should do what they have done, and that all other *solutions* are wrong.

As I have moved through my own experiences around the addition or subtraction of various foods or supplements, I am often engaged by other people as to my advice on the merits of one style of eating over another, and the DOs and DON'Ts that come with each modality.

Many people feel that, because I have been so successful with moving disease out of my body, that I have all the answers. I would like to state categorically here that *there is no one way to eat.* All is experience. What works for one person, may not necessarily work for another. All are on their own path, choosing the experiences that best move their soul forward.

An overall view of food as a source of energy is the best model to work with, and I came to understand this more as I moved through my own healing experience. At first, I was very strict with myself, and this worked very well for me because I *believed* whole-heartedly in what I was doing. I felt it would work, and it did. I was very impressed with the macrobiotic diet and the results it yielded for me. It would be my strongest recommendation. It has a great track record. Also, I approached which methods I would use for myself mostly from a *feeling* of which ones were best for me. I allowed my guidance to direct me. I also used common sense. From an energy standpoint, it does not make sense to me that meat harvested from animals who are caged in large facilities that never see the light of day—who are so constricted by space that they have no ability to even move about while being surrounded by their own feces and who are pumped full of antibiotics and fed pesticide ridden food—was a wise choice for consumption. The energy of these animals is of a particularly low vibration.

Many animals do come to earth to be used as a food source. They have agreed to this. What they have not agreed to is the deplorable lack of respect for their important contribution to the service of mankind at this time in our planet's history. Far better to eat an ethically raised animal or a wild animal who willingly gives its life so that humans may survive on the planet at this time. In many cultures from the past, animals were always honored when they were taken for food during a hunt. These civilizations understood the natural *give and take* between the animal kingdom and the human kingdom—and respected the sacrifice. No ones ever really dies, they just transform. Animals are no different than humans in this regard. It would be ethical to allow animals to have a more enjoy-able ride through the third dimensional reality, and I am sure the animals would like to be more respected at this time.

One must be discerning around what resonates with them when it comes to eating modalities. So while I do not eat meat, that does not mean there is anything wrong with eating meat. It is a choice. And your choices around food can change. They will. I found that, as time went on, I was holding some fears around eating certain things. I would never have anything with sugar, alcohol, dairy, or meat in it. This served me well in the early days while I was trying to understand the overarching reason for my illness. These foods, energetically, are of a lower vibration. They feed cancer cells. Since all is vibration or frequency, my goal was to raise my vibration to a point where illness could no longer be sustained. So I was very diligent in that effort. Now that my body is clean, and cancer finds it an inhospitable place to reside, I can allow myself to eat foods with these substances in them, without the fear that was accompanying me in the earlier days. I only eat them in small quantities, however; as I find I love how energetic and awesome I feel when I eat higher vibrational foods.

Right out of the garden and into your mouth is the freshest and highest nutrition, and after that, anything that gets you the closest to that is the most desired. I love berry season in my neck of the woods. I can literally walk out my door in August and September and pick wild raspberries, blueberries and blackberries off the vine and then put them on my breakfast cereal or in a salad. This is as good as it gets! And remember to thank the earth each time you take something she willingly and lovingly supplies for you. Eating is one of the most sensual pleasures given to us at this time. Enjoy your food!! That is the best advice I can give you.

Breaking Patterns

Patterns are doing the same thing in the same way, day after day. Lifetime after lifetime. The new consciousness revolution is about doing things a different way. Breaking new ground. Stepping out of the herd and being fearless in your approach to life. Changing how you think. Who you are. What you want.

Patterns keep you locked into a repetitive reality that deals you the same experience over and over again—albeit with different people and different circumstances—the underlying energy is always repeated. I have noticed how much easier it is to spot other people's patterns now that I have more awareness around this. I am getting better at seeing my own patterns as well, but your own are a little harder to see, as you are more emotionally invested in your own patterns just as others are in theirs, and so it is always easier to see someone else's more clearly than your own.

I have a friend who has created situations of betrayal her entire life. When she was younger she felt ostracized from her family because they seemed to always put her last—or this is how she felt. She encountered the same experience with friends, who would stab her in the back when she least expected it. A husband who betrayed her with other women over and over again. Family members would again strike out at her when she was only trying to get closer to them. This was a reoccurring theme in her life. As she became more aware, she realized this and so she started doing things differently.

Acknowledging that she created her reality, and accepting that she was feeling these deep feelings of betrayal, she noticed she would start feeling like a victim around these people who she felt were betraying her. She allowed the feelings of hurt to come up within her. She felt them deeply. She then allowed herself to let go of any expectations around how she felt others should be treating her. She let go of worrying about what anyone thought of her and started loving herself for who she was. All of the drama and heartfelt trauma she had been experiencing just dissolved. She now feels nothing but love for all of the people. This pattern has no more emotional hooks to draw her in—she has transmuted the energy that she was holding onto deep in her heart and soul.

This was obviously a very deep pattern that had been manifesting in many lifetimes, and wanting to be let go of this time around—this is a time of completion for many of us here on the planet. This is an example of how healing can take place. The physical body responds each time you transmute fear in your cells. This allows for a higher vibration of love to move into your body.

Breaking patterns can be as difficult as the one I described above, or it can be as simple as just being aware and committing to doing something different every day. Buy different types of food. Order something you have never ordered at a restaurant. Walk a different way to work. Drive to a town you have never visited before. Talk to someone you have never met. Think new thoughts. Find something you are strongly opinionated about and look at the other side of the argument. Take up a hobby that you know nothing about. Change it up in any and every way possible. Step outside your comfort zone at least once a day.

Breaking patterns always means doing something that does not feel easy or familiar. This is how you create new energy pathways. This is how the universe can send you miraculous things you have always been wanting. This is how your life changes. Be fearless. Have fun. Be the *you* who is wanting to come through!

Chapter 35.
THE ROLE OF CANCER SOCIETIES/RESEARCH

I struggled with whether I should speak to this subject, and after much weighing and contemplation, I felt I should. You see, I get so many people call me who have either been diagnosed with cancer themselves or who have a loved one who has been diagnosed with cancer. They are usually pretty upset, very fearful, and are looking to me for advice on how they can save themselves. They are afraid of the prospect of chemotherapy and radiation. They are being told this is their only option. They have heard that I have done something different and have been successful and they want to know what I have done so I can impart it to them.

If you are this far along in the book, you know by now that it is a long story and not one that can be imparted in a few minutes on the telephone. The magic bullet is this: *The power of healing comes from within oneself. It does not come from outside circumstances.*

The cancer societies say they are searching for a cure for cancer. I think I would be correct in saying that this is their overarching mandate. The one that gets the most press. I realize that they also fund many other aspects of cancer care. I personally would like to see some changes in the way they fund new research and initiatives. I would like to tell you about my experience with the cancer society in my city. This story takes place long before I was personally diagnosed with cancer.

When my daughters started junior high school, I heard many people discussing the increased rates of smoking among young girls. This concerned me, and I started looking into it. I found that yes, it was on the rise, and I felt compelled to try and do something to address this. I happen to come upon a campaign started in the southern United States, called *The Truth Campaign.*

The state of Florida sued the tobacco industry for targeting youth in their ads, and won. They received many millions of dollars and decided to put this money into a program to help stop young people from taking up smoking. They did this by going into the schools at the junior high level and educating the kids about how they were being hoodwinked by these big tobacco giants into smoking. You see, the savvy marketing companies that were hired to do this knew from their research that young people engage in risk-taking behavior at this age. They like to rebel. So they decided to use reverse psychology and encourage the students to rebel against the tobacco giants. They did this by giving them pen, paint, paper and canvas and asked them to design advertisements that spoke back to the advertisements that the tobacco industry was using to entice them. This was brilliant. They rolled this out over the whole state, and huge prizes were to be won by the students who came up with the best ads. These ads were put up all over the school walls, and the students themselves voted for the best ones.

The most publicized winning ad was one that showed a picture of the Marlborough brand which shows three cowboys riding horses. The winning ad showed the three horses, just like the original, only instead of men in the saddle, there were three body bags. A profound visual statement. These student ads were placed in major magazines and received huge public awareness. Unfortunately, the tobacco industry, who were being sued in various other states at that time, settled with the other states only if they would agree not to run truth campaigns. It was a short-lived but spectacular success.

I saw no reason to reinvent the wheel and decided that we could run our own little truth campaign locally. It had proven itself after all.

I approached the principal of the school and he loved it. A wonderful man he was. Very supportive. Now my part was to come up with the funding for this project. I was sure that preventing youth from smoking and by extension preventing lung cancer was a great thing. I felt sure the cancer society would love this initiative, and be happy to partner with the school. The principal and a local nurse practitioner felt it would be a great pilot project that we could roll out to other schools possibly all across the country, such was the level of our enthusiasm. I asked the cancer society for help, thinking that they would love to partner with a plan that could effectively help reduce smoking levels potentially all across the country.

The cancer society told me that they did not fund initiatives at the community level, but they would be happy to give us pieces of paper commending the kids for their efforts. I was pretty shocked and disappointed. The amount of money that gets raised at the community level and given to such organizations is huge. I asked the heart foundation. Received the same answer. So this was my experience, and I realize I cannot paint all of them with the same brush, however, there is something fundamentally wrong here. Have they gotten so large that they cannot see the forest for the trees? Is there something I am missing here?

I can assure you that we ran a very successful truth campaign without the help of either of these organizations. I received money from our local hospital foundation, and from local business people. All of them had a vested interest in seeing this unfold, for they all had children in the school. We ran the campaign for two years. On the third year, the principal changed and the new one did not see the benefit in continuing it. There was a follow up done a few years later and the number of youths who started smoking from that group of junior high students was significantly lower than other years. I feel strongly that community level initiatives have a high rate of effectiveness and should be given more attention.

So my question is this: *Has cancer become big business?* I think there is merit to this question. There is a lot of money being made off of sick people. And more and more people are getting sick. I remember hearing the author Richard Beliveau (*Foods that Fight Cancer*) mention that he develops chemotherapy drugs from studying plants and so he felt ethically compelled to write a book about the value of eating these foods—he considered them to be natural chemotherapy. How much money would be made in the pharmaceutical industry by telling people to eat these foods?

There is a wonderfully explicit and shocking movie that has garnered millions of views on YouTube. In this documentary the producers show how they methodically researched what is actually going on in the world with the suppression of free energy, medical cures, and other such mind-blowing tactics that are being directed from the highest levels of a global elite upon an unsuspecting world. The scope of their revelations is difficult for the average person to comprehend.

The desire at the end of this educational piece of work is to accept the status quo and move into a world with new solutions and positive thinking. I really encourage people to watch this in its entirety. I was astounded at how much of this research had come to me intuitively. It is called "Thrive" and you can see more about their movement by going to their site at www.thrivemovement.com.

It seems to me that, if you really want to cure illness of any sort, you should start looking at healthy people, not sick people. I am reminded of one of Einstein's famous quotes:"We cannot solve our problems with the same level of thinking that created them."

It seems to me that people are being helped to be sick longer by all of the drugs they are prescribed. There are certainly situations where people need and are helped by pharmaceutical remedies; I am not speaking about those situations. The increase of prescription drug addiction is pandemic. Who is gaining from this? Certainly not the everyday person. These large organizations are being given huge amounts of money from everyday people who are fund raising for cures to help their loved ones. Since they have not found a cure to date, perhaps people like me are the model that they can study that will provide the cure. There are many stories more miraculous than mine of people who have defied the odds of what the medical scientific communities think their outcome should have been.

Anita Moorjani comes to mind. You can read her miraculous story in her book *Dying To Be Me*. It is the real life story of a woman who was taken to the hospital with her organs shutting down—on the brink of death after four years of cancer—and her miraculous recovery against all medical odds. To find out more about her you can visit her site at www. anitamoorjani.com.

Or you can read about the medical miracle experienced by Dr. Eben Alexander, a neurosurgeon who contracted an extremely rare illness that shut down his neocortex putting him into a deep coma for seven days. During his coma he journeyed beyond this world and communed with the divine source of the universe itself. Previous to this life altering experience, he advocated near death experiences were simply fantasies produced by the brain under stress. Today he believes the soul is real and that death is not the end of personal existence but only a transition. You can visit him at www.lifebeyonddeath.net.

There is also a young man named Chris Wark who was diagnosed with Stage III colon cancer at the age of twenty-six. He had surgery and then was told he needed nine months of chemotherapy. He wasn't too sure about this, so looked into what this entailed and saw that it would totally crash his immune system. As a result of this information, he decided to look into various alternative treatments and found that the raw food movement was having success, so mentioned this to his doctor. His doctor told him not to do this, as it would interfere with his chemo-therapy. He felt something was inherently wrong with that advice, so he decided to pursue his own path with alternative solutions. He is still here today, and you can read his wonderful story and more about his life since cancer by going to www.chrisbeatcancer.com.

Study *these* people. I was once told by a scientific-minded person that I was only a control group of one. I did not fit the criteria for scientific study due to my lonely number. So when I say study people like myself and others like me, I am thinking outside the established scientific research protocols. The ones that allow only doctors and scientists with university credentials, specialized institutionally condoned education, and industry publication endorsements, to be the only ones deemed worthy of contributing to the search for a cure. After all the money and all the clinical controls that are in place, where are the results? Where is the cure?

It seems to me that there is more effort being put into managing illness by treating the symptoms of illness. Again I am prompted to quote Einstein:

"Insanity is doing the same thing over and over and expecting a different outcome."

In the early days of my cancer, I allowed the medical profession to do it their way, I allowed them to pump me full of dyes and harmful substances to study my body and to see if the cancer had spread. After the first bout—and three days of a nasty rash—I decided that would be the last time I allowed this. I had gone to great lengths to clean up my body at this point, and I felt this sort of study and diagnosis was not in my best interest.

At the end of three years—and due to the success of all that I have done—I believe I have the right to say it would be highly appropriate to look into studying the new ways that are being undertaken by those of us who are willing to do something different. Ask us what we've done. Listen and then apply our methodology in a research model that approaches outcomes in a less invasive and less damaging way. There is no need to cut us open, or pump us full of dyes or radioactive isotopes to understand what we are doing and see the wisdom in it. I will say again.

Study people like me and others like me, and you will find amazing new information.

It is now the time to broaden our idea of how research is conducted. Science has become no better than religion for dogmatic rules. The dollar is more worshipped than the human quality of life. We are all aware of this, and each of us has the responsibility to stand up and demand that new choices be made available to us. Period. I would like to stress that I do not speak of the everyday people who work in the front lines of the healthcare industry and in organizations like the cancer society. I know these caring souls are doing the best work they can for all of the people they are trying to help. I am speaking to the individuals who are at the top of the pyramid. If your thoughts create your reality, and I believe this to be a true statement, then mass thoughts create mass reality. It is incumbent on each individual to clearly send their desire to see change in how our medical industry is responding to the needs of this time.

As I see it—and have experienced it—there is a very large disconnect between the traditional Western predominately science minded health-care community and the new age, metaphysical, alternative, holistic, and natural healing community. I would love nothing more than to have them work in unison for the benefit of all humankind.

Summary

Three years later, as I finish writing the closing lines of my comprehensive experience into healing and cancer, I am sure many are wondering what my state of health is at this point. Am I cancer free?

Since everyone has cancer cells in their body, it would be incorrect for anyone to say they are cancer free. However, here is where I am at. The cancer never spread from my breast to any other part of my body after the original traveling parts were removed by the psychic surgeon.

I am in total and complete remission. I can feel that there is no active cancer in my body at this point. As for the large mass that once filled my entire breast – it is almost completely gone. It does take some time for the body to absorb such a large mass, but it is doing so very quickly now. I feel fantastic. I am told often that I look healthy, almost like I have a *glow* about me. I never tire of hearing these lovely unsolicited validations of my efforts in healing myself.

Books That Have Found Me

The following books are listed here so that the reader may indulge personally if they so choose to read some of the mind-expanding literature that found its way to me at what seemed to be the most perfect time. Each of these books contributed to the healing of my body, mind and spirit. Remember that if anything in whatever book you read does not resonate with you, simply let it go.

References

Alexander, Eben. *Proof of Heaven.* A Neurosurgeon's Journey. Simon & Schuster, 2012.

Anka, Darryl. *Bashar Blueprint for Change:* A Message from our Future. New Solutions Publishing, Dec 1, 1990.

Beliveau, Richard. *Foods That Fight Cancer.* Essential Foods to Help Prevent Cancer. DK Publishing, 2007.

Braden, Gregg. *The God Code:* The Secret of Our Past, the Promise of Our Future. Hay House, Incorporated, 2004.

Bryan, Jessica. *Psychic Surgery & Faith Healing*: An Exploration of Multi-Dimensional Realities, Indigenous Healing, and Medical Miracles in the Philippine Lowlands. Red Wheel, 2008.

Cannon, Dolores. *Between Death and Life*: Conversations With A Spirit. Dolores Cannon, 1993.

Carey, Ken. *The Starseed Transmissions*. Harper Collins Paperback Edition, 1991.

Carroll, Lee. *Kryon*. www.kryon.com

Chopra, Deepak. *Life after Death*: The Burden of Proof. Three Rivers Press, Crown Publishing Group, a Division of Random House Inc. New York. 2006.

Cori, Patricia. *Atlantis Rising*: The Struggle of Darkness and Light. North Atlantic Books, May 18, 2010.

Crawford, April. *In The Afterlife*. Connecting Wave, 2011.

Dyer, Wayne W. *The Shift*: Taking Your Life from Ambition to Meaning. Hay House, Inc, Mar 1, 2010.

Eadie, Betty J. *Embraced by the Light*. Random House LLC, 1994.

Haich, Elisabeth. *Initiation*. Aurora Press, Incorporated, 2000.

Hand-Clow, Barbara. *The Alchemy of Nine Dimensions*: The 2011/2012 Prophecies and Nine Dimensions of Consciousness. Hampton Roads Publishing, Apr 1, 2010.

Hay, Louise. *You Can Heal Your Life*. Accessible Publishing Systems, 2008.

Hicks, Ester and Jerry. *Ask and it is Given*: Learning to Manifest Your Desires. Accessible Publishing Systems, 2008.

Kagan, Annie. *The Afterlife of Billy Fingers:* How My Bad Boy Brother Proved to Me There's Life After Death. (2013) Hampton Roads Publishing Inc.

Lipton, Bruce H. *The Biology of Belief:* Unleashing The Power of Consciousness, Matter and Miracles. Mountain of Love Productions, 2008.

Marciniak, Barbara. *Family of Light:* Pleiadian Tales and Lessons in Living. Inner Traditions / Bear & Co, Jan 14, 2011.

McTaggart, Lynne. *The Intention Experiment.* Using Your Thoughts to Change Your Life and the World. Simon and Schuster, Jan 9, 2007.

Melchizedek, Drunvalo. *The Serpent of Light:* Beyond 2012. Weiser Books, Jan 1, 2008.

Milanovich, Norma J. *We, The Arcturians.* Athena Publishing, 1990.

Millman, Dan. *The Way of the Peaceful Warrior:* A Book That Changes Lives. New World Library, 1980.

Mitchell, Stephen. *Tao Te Ching:* Persona. HarperCollins, Aug 28, 1992.

Newton, Michael. *Journey of Souls.* Llewellyn Worldwide, Sep 1, 2010.

Roberts, Jane. *Seth Speaks.* Amber-Allen Publishing, Apr 1, 2012.

Rasha. *Onesness.* Earthstar Press, Jan 1, 2008.

Packer, Sanaya Roman Duane. *Opening to Channel:* How to Connect with your Guide. H. J. Kramer Incorporated, Apr 1, 1987.

Prakasha, Padma Aon. *The Christ Blueprint:* 13 Keys to Christ Consciousness. North Atlantic Books, 2010.

Priest, Lyssa Royal Keith. *The Prism of Lyra:* An Exploration of Human Galactic Heritage. Light Technology Publishing, Mar 1, 2011.

Schucman, Helen, Thetford, William T. *A Course in Miracles.* Course in Miracles Society, 2009.

Shadyac, Tom. *Life's Operating Manual:* With The Fear and Truth Dialogues. Hay House Incorporated, Apr 22, 2013.

Sitchin, Zecharia. *The Stairway to Heaven*: Book II of the Earth Chronicles. HarperCollins, Apr 1, 1999.

Solara. *11:11*: Inside The Doorway. Star-Borne Unlimited, Sep 1, 1992.

Starr, Jelaila. *We are the Nibiruans*: Return of the 12th Planet. Nibiruan Council, 2004.

Tolle, Eckhart. *The Power of Now*: A Guide to Spiritual Enlightenment. New World Library, 1999.

Troyer, Patricia. *Crystal Personalities:* A Quick Reference to Special Forms of Quartz (Crystals and New Age) (1995) Stone People Publishing Company.

Walsch, Neale Donald. *Conversations With God*: An Uncommon Dialogue. Penguin, Oct 29, 1996.

Williamson, Marianne. *Woman's Worth*: A Return to Love. Random House LLC, Jan 23, 2013.

Zimmerman, Lauren. *Called*. Volume I of Other Worlds. Lauren Zimmerman, Dec 4, 2010.

Zukav, Gary. *The Seat of the Soul*. Simon and Schuster, Jun 19, 2007.

Documentaries and Movies

The following movies and documentaries I found to be highly enlightening. They can be accessed for the most part on the internet. Just put them into Google and sites where they can be viewed or purchased will come up.

What the Bleep do we Know *by Feature Film*

Black Whole *by Nassim Haramein*

Zeitgeist - The Movie 2007

Zeitgeist - Addendum 2008

Zeitgeist - Moving Forward 2011

Spirit Science – (available on YouTube) *by Jordan Duchnycz*

Sirius - The Movie